Back Stretching

Back strengthening and stretching exercises for everyone

By David Nordmark

Copyright © 2012 By David Nordmark

Disclaimer

The exercises and advice contained within this course may be too strenuous or dangerous for some people, and the reader(s) should consult a physician before engaging in them. The author and publisher of this course are not responsible in any manner whatsoever for any injury which may occur through reading and following the instructions herein.

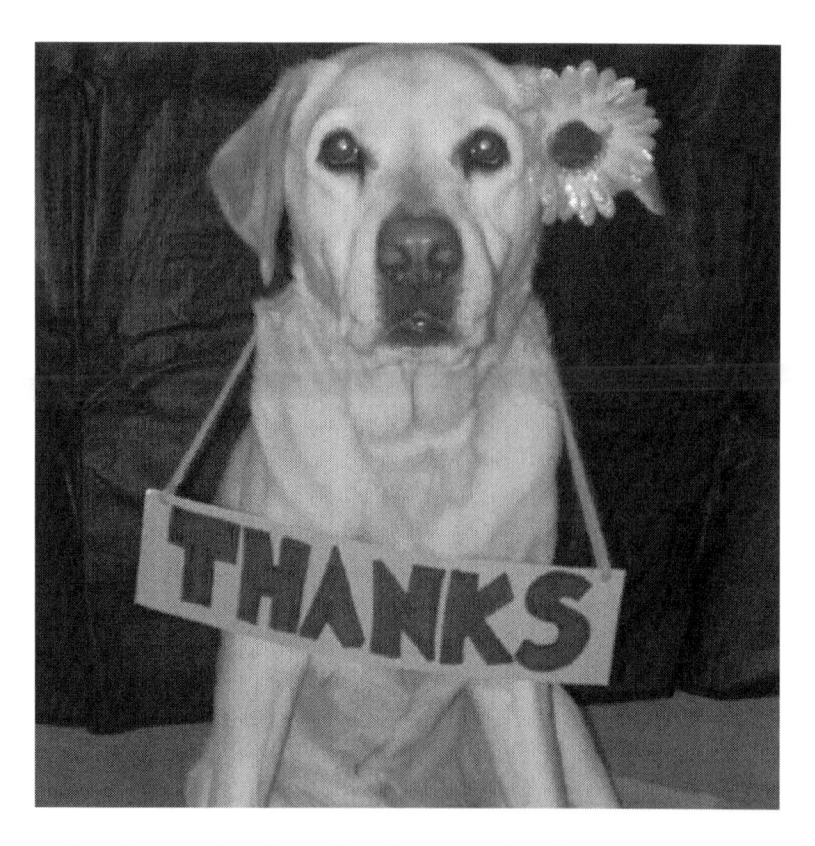

Thank-you for downloading my book. Please REVIEW my book on Amazon. I appreciate your feedback so that I can make the next version even better. Thank-you so much!

Table Of Contents

Why We Suffer From Back Pain   6
What Is The Secret Of Back Pain Relief?   8
A Few Notes On The Back Bridge   9
Isometric Neck Exercises   10
How To Stretch   12

Back Stretching Exercises

Secretary Stretch   16
Shoulder Blade Pinch   18
Lower Back Flattener   20
Elongation Stretch   22
Knee To Shoulder Stretch   23
Double Knee To Chest Stretch   24
Lower Back And Hip Stretch   25
Reaching Upper Back Stretch   26
Kneeling Back Arch Stretch   28
Standing Back Rotation Stretch   30
Spinal Twist   32
Squat Stretch   34
Cobra Stretch   35

Hamstring Stretch	36
Lying Groin Stretch	38
Neck Stretch	39
4 Point Neck Stretch	40
"Praying" Stretch	42
Cross Shoulder Stretch	44
Back Shoulder Stretch	46
Straight Arm Stretch	48
Straight Arm Behind Back Stretch	50
Cross Over Shoulder Stretch	52
Standing Waist Stretch	54
Bent-Over Upper Back Stretch	56
Table Maker Stretch	58
Dynamic Bridging Stretch	60

Back Strengthening Exercises

Grounded Back Twist	62
Sumo Squat Stretch	64
Sumo Squat Kicks	66
Ying/Yang Bends	68
Tai Chi Waist Turner	70
Gymnastic Shoulder Shrugs	72
Gymnastic Shoulder Pulls	74
Gymnastic Shoulder Pulls 2	76

Towel Pulls	78
Side Towel Pulls	80
Dynamic Lion Stretch	82
Kneeling Back Bend	84
Forward Rows	86
Hand Supported Back Bridge	88
Floor Bow Posture	90
Wall Walking	92
The Table Maker	94
The Stretcher	96
Reverse Leg Lifts	98
Torso Lifts	100

Isometric Neck Exercises

Reverse Neck Contraction	102
Forward Neck Contraction	105
Side Neck Contraction (left to right)	108
Side Neck Contraction (right to left)	111
Suggested Back Stretching And Strengthening Routines	114
Intramuscular Stimulation	116
About the Author	122

About the Models   122

One Last Thing   124

Why We Suffer From Back Pain

It is almost inevitable. At some point each and every one one of us will experience back pain. Hurting your back is just about the worst injury you can sustain. If you injure your arm or leg, you can still hobble around and get things done. With your back, not so much. When you hurt your back you turn into an old man or woman overnight. Simply getting out of bed can be a chore. Simple tasks like sitting in a chair or walking become impossible.

Whether it's feeling a twinge after raking the leaves or the discomfort we experience after sitting in a chair all day, back pain is something we've all experienced. It affects the old and the young, the out of shape and the hyper fit (although the former more than the latter, obviously).

Why is this? Why is chronic back pain such an issue, particularly in western societies?

Some of the more commonly accepted factors are that we live much more sedentary lifestyles, we get too little exercise, and many of us are overweight. These are undoubtedly all true. A large percentage of the modern population spends their working day sitting in chairs, which is extremely hard on the back. Lack of exercise leads to weak muscles while every pound of extra weight puts added strain on the spine. None of this is helpful.

Despite the fact that all of the above are true, they're not the most important source of back pain.

What is then?

It comes down to evolution. Our backs are literally structurally unsound from the get go. Here's why.

There is nothing elegant about the process of evolution. Evolution is a process by which existing systems are adapted to take advantage of new situations. In the case of the human back the spine was originally developed to support an even weight along its full length. This worked fantastically when we walked in one way or another on all four limbs. When we began to walk upright this all changed. A system that was perfectly adapted to working parallel to the ground now had to work perpendicular to it. This is the true root of our back pain issues.

Think about it this way. Imagine a tall, thin flagpole. Got it? Now place an enormous weight right on top of it. What is going to happen to it? A flagpole simply isn't designed to support a large weight. It is going to bend and sway under the weight. Most of the strain will be felt at the flagpole's base. You don't have to be an engineer to understand that this structure is fundamentally unsound.

In many ways the human spine resembles that flagpole. It is a pole on which a large weight (our head) is placed. Can you see why so many people suffer from back pain, especially lower back pain? Thanks to the wondrous process of evolution, we're almost designed for it.

Compounding this problem (beyond the already mentioned lack of exercise and weight issues) is that so many of us live sedentary lives sitting in chairs. The unnatural act of "chair sitting" (we didn't evolve sitting in chairs for hours at a time) means that we are constantly bending our backs forwards for huge amounts of time throughout the day. Our backs are designed to move in every direction, backwards, forwards, and side to side. However, people rarely give their backs an opportunity to do so. The result of this preponderance of forward bending is that stress builds up in our back muscles with no chance for release. This is also a source of a great deal of back pain.

What Is The Secret Of Back Pain Relief?

Having said all of this, what is the secret of real back pain relief? In a few words, back bending. From my experience with back pain, performing exercises and stretches that bend the back backwards are the single most effective thing you can do to have a healthy back. There are many other stretches that are included in this book which also help strengthen and release the tension in the back muscles. However, I've found that back bending exercises are by far the most effective.

The other important area to exercise, which most books ignore, are the neck muscles. The neck muscles are your first line of defense in supporting your head. When people have weak neck muscles their heads typically lean forward. Aside from causing additional strain on the spine, this can also lead to other conditions such as migraines and headaches. The most dramatic example of the potential negative effects of weak neck muscles can be seen in the elderly. Often if you observe a senior citizen walking around you may observe that he or she has a hunched back and poor posture. This is usually the result of weak neck muscles over time. What happens is that weak neck muscles allow the head to lean forward. If this condition is not stopped the head then drags the shoulders forward, and later the upper back. The result is the stooped posture seen among too many of our senior citizens. Don't let this entirely preventable condition happen to you. Work on developing strong back and neck muscles today.

A Few Notes On The Back Bridge

The Back Bridge is an exercise used by both gymnasts and wrestlers to build strong, healthy backs. From my experience it is the best exercise you can do to strengthen and stretch your back. It is an advanced exercise, but with patience and practice anyone can perform it. It can be performed as a stretch by gently rocking back and forth (see the Dynamic Bridging Stretch) or as a stretch and strengthening exercise by holding it for time (see the Hand Supported Back Bridge). I completely understand how intimidating this exercise looks at first. Most people are not used to bending their backs backwards at all, never mind like this. Plus the fact that you have to bend your neck as well is a little, well, scary.

Those were my exact thoughts when I attempted to perform the back bridge the first time. When I initially arched my back I actually heard little snaps all along my spine, kind of like twigs snapping. However, although I was only able to do it for a few seconds, it felt good. When it comes to strengthening your spine, torso, and neck, it really can't be beat. If you are intimidated, I highly suggest you perform some of the easier back bending exercises, like the Cobra. However, as you master the easier exercises and stretches and start to feel more confident, you will want to give the back bridge a try. Once you can do it you will know that your neck and spine are stronger and healthier than 99% of the people out there.

Isometric Neck Exercises

Now, like I've said, increasing the strength of your neck muscles is vitally important to having a strong and healthy spine. The absolutely best exercise for this, as I've already stated, is some version of the back bridge. However, this exercise is advanced, and most people understandably don't want to attempt it right off the bat. This is why I've included some isometric neck exercises for beginners. This will allow you to build strength in your neck without having to contort yourself into a bridge.

Isometrics work on the principle of self-resistance. When you exert muscular force against an immovable object, it is a scientific fact that you will get stronger. The process by which this happens is known as an isometric contraction. Here's how it works.

Imagine you pick up a paper cup. In order to do so, your brain activates a few muscle fibers in order to accomplish that task. It doesn't activate all of them as this would be overkill, and your body is always trying to conserve energy. Now, imagine you try to move something large, like your house. Can you move it? Of course not. However, your brain doesn't know this and is willing to give it a try. At first it will activate a few muscle fibers, just like it does for the paper cup. However, when no movement occurs your brain will quickly activate more and more muscle fibers until all of them are being used. If this is done repeatedly overtime, your brain will actually grow more muscle fibers in an attempt to accomplish this impossible task. That's how static contractions can be used to build and strengthen muscle, and it is this principle that you can use to build your neck muscles.

When performing a static contraction, the key thing is to focus on your breath through 3 phases. As you slowly increase the muscle tension you will want to breath in through you nose for 3 to 4 seconds. At this point the contraction should be at its most powerful. You will now want to exhale through your mouth for 7 to 10 seconds. As you do so press your tongue to the roof of your mouth so that you make an almost snakelike "SSSSSSS" sound. At the end of the contraction you will want to slowly release the tension for 3 to 4 seconds by again breathing in through you nose. This is the breathing pattern you should follow at all times. At no time should you hold your breath for any reason. The act of breathing out or in allows you to control your blood pressure. Holding your breath robs you of this ability, and you could potentially faint or worse. Always remember; never hold your breath when performing isometric exercises of any kind!

How To Stretch

When stretching or performing any of the exercises in this book, it is vital that you do it with a happy and relaxed mind. Most people, when they stretch, do the exact opposite. They don't like stretching, so they approach it as a chore. They grimace and scrunch up their face as they attempt to work their tight muscles. What happens? They make little progress and often wind up injuring themselves.

The reason for this is that when you exercise or stretch with an angry mind, your brain is sending out angry signals to your muscles as well. This tightens them and actually winds up working against you. Do not do this.

Rather, you should look forward to stretching. Look at it as a calming and relaxing experience. Breathe deeply, and move gently into the stretch. You will want to feel a gentle stretch, but nothing more. Never force anything. You should never stretch to the point of pain. If you do, back off. When you stretch too far your mind sends signals to your muscles to contract in an effort to avoid injury. This is not what you want. Rather, you want to hold a gentle stretch for time. You want to feel a slight tension in your muscles that then slowly dissipates once your brain is convinced that there is no chance for injury. As you stretch use your brain as well. Visualize your muscles in your mind's eye and tell them to relax. Remember, your brain controls your muscles. Make sure you make use of it!

How To Perform The Stretching Exercises In This Book

In the back of the book I have listed back stretching and strengthening routines for beginner, intermediate, and advanced levels. If you are a beginner, I suggest you start with these. However, these routines are not written in stone. When you get more comfortable, I suggest you try to make up your own routines, depending on how you feel. Try all of the stretches and exercises listed in this book at least once. Undoubtedly you will find some you really like, and others you don't care for. Some will be ineffective, whereas others will just hit the right spot. It is hard to say which ones are which as we are all different. However, once you learn which ones feel good to you, try making up your own routines. It isn't very hard. Start off with a few stretches to warm up and then move onto some of the back strengthening exercises. You know your body better than anyone else. Listen to your body at all times, and you really can't go wrong.

Back Stretching Exercises

Secretary Stretch

This movement will provide a nice stretch for your lower back, side, and the top of the hip. Your upper back, back of head, shoulders, and elbows should remain flat on the floor at all times.

1. Lie flat on your back with your knees bent and together and your feet flat on the floor. Interlace your fingers and place them behind your head.
2. Bring your left knee over your right leg.
3. Use your left leg to gently pull your right leg towards the floor. You should feel a good stretch along the side of your hip and in your lower back. Hold the stretch for 30 seconds while breathing calmly and slowly.

Do not try and force your right leg down so that it touches the floor. Only bring it down as far as you need to in order to feel a relaxing stretch. Repeat with the other side, crossing your right leg over your left and bringing it down to the floor.

17

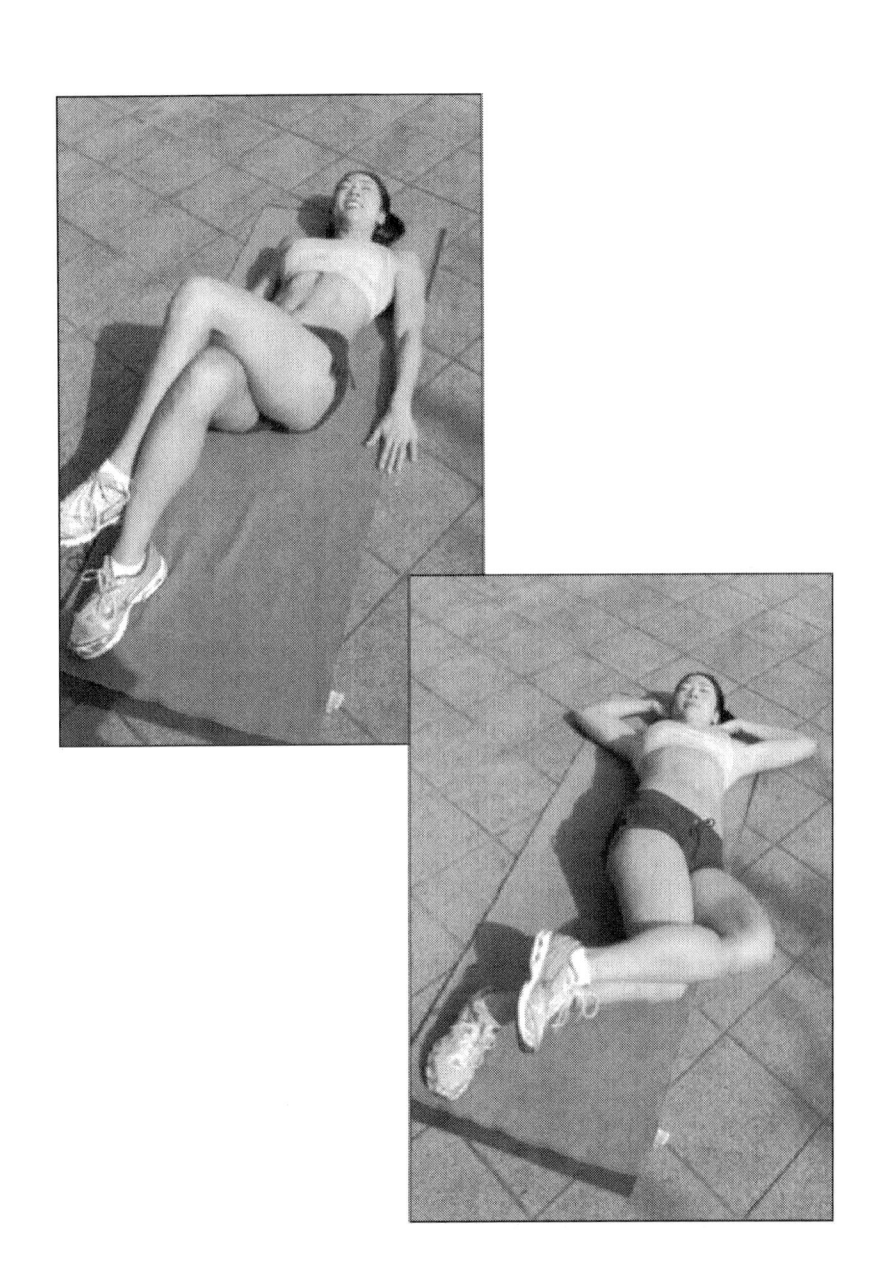

Shoulder Blade Pinch

This exercise reduces tension in the upper back and will help you perform other neck stretches like the Neck Stretch.

1. Lie flat on your back with your knees bent and your fingers interlaced behind your head.
2. Pull your shoulder blades together. If you perform this pinching motion correctly your chest should rise.

Hold the tension for 3 to 5 seconds and repeat 3 - 4 times.

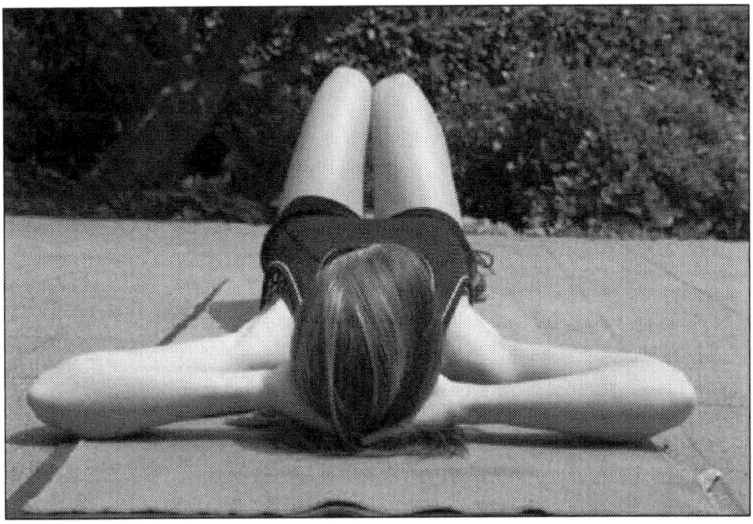

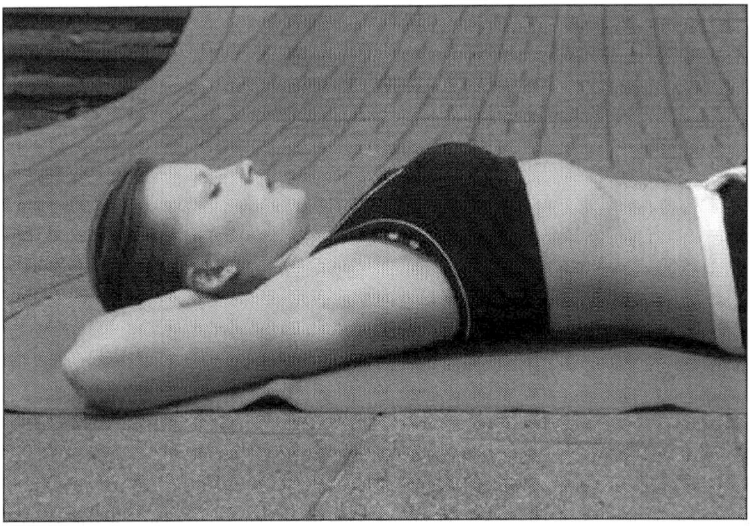

Lower Back Flattener

This exercise relieves tension in the lower back while simultaneously tightening your gluteus (butt) and abdominal muscles.

1. Begin from a bent knee position with your hands interlaced behind your head.
2. Flex and tighten your abdominal muscles for 5 to 8 seconds.
3. Your goal is to lower your back flat to the ground, if possible.

As your perform this exercise focus on maintaining an even and steady tension in your stomach. Repeat 2 to 3 times.

21

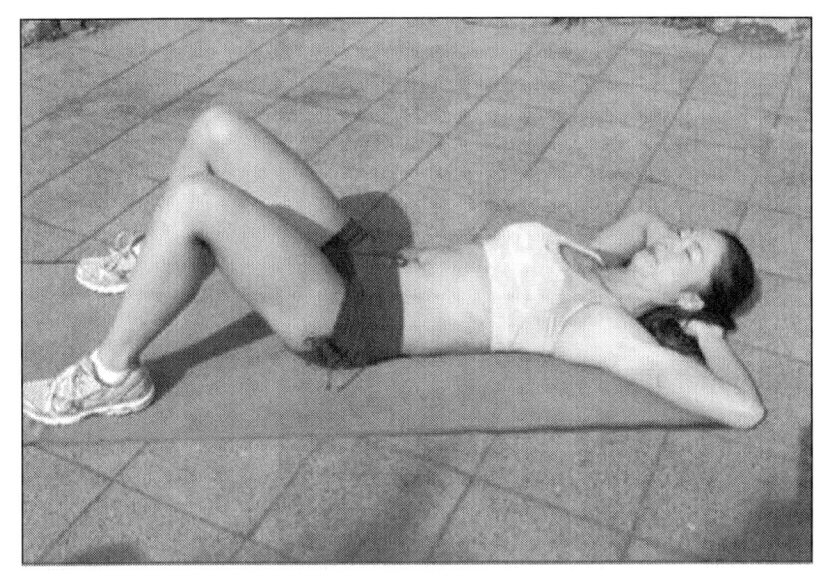

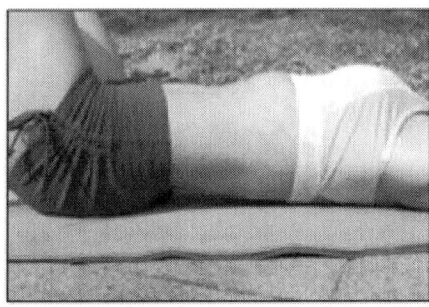

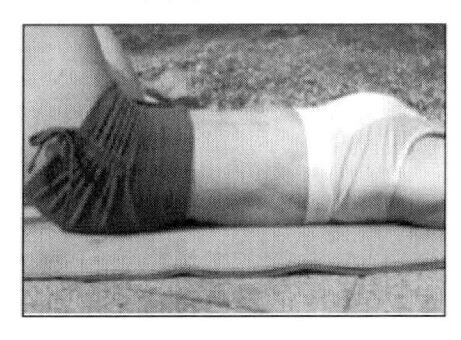

Elongation Stretch

This simple stretch not only works your back, but your entire body as well.

1. Lie flat on your back with your toes pointed and your arms above your head, palms facing upwards.
2. Stretch your toes and palms in opposite directions. Breathe in and hold this stretch for 5 seconds, then relax.

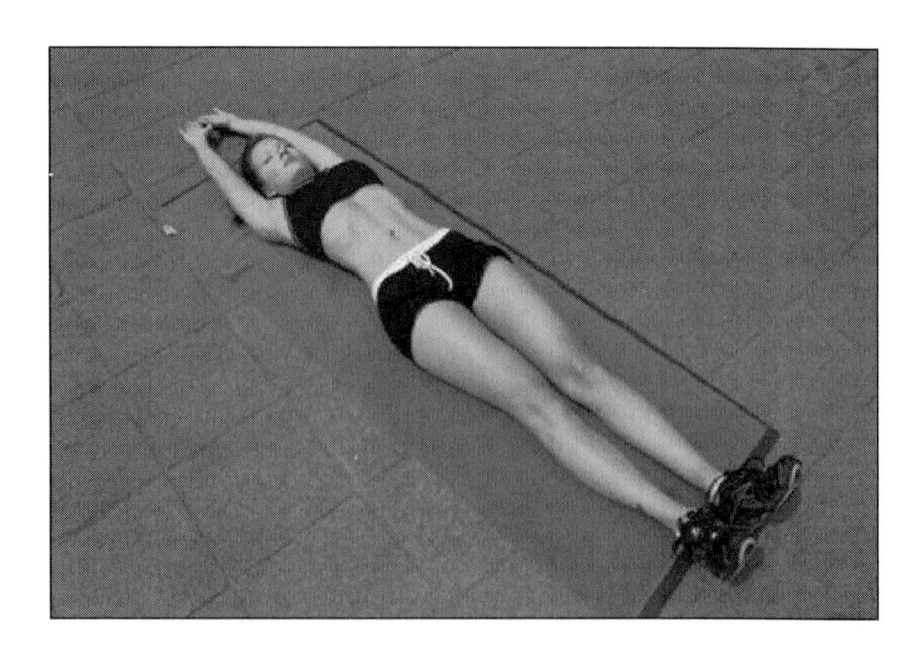

Knee To Shoulder Stretch

This stretch works your lower back as well as your legs and feet.

1. Lie flat on your back.
2. Bring your right knee towards your shoulder, avoiding your rib cage. Clasp your fingers just below the knee.
3. Gently pull your knee towards your right shoulder.

Hold this stretch 30 seconds. Focus on keeping your lower back flat on the floor as your perform this movement. Repeat with your left leg.

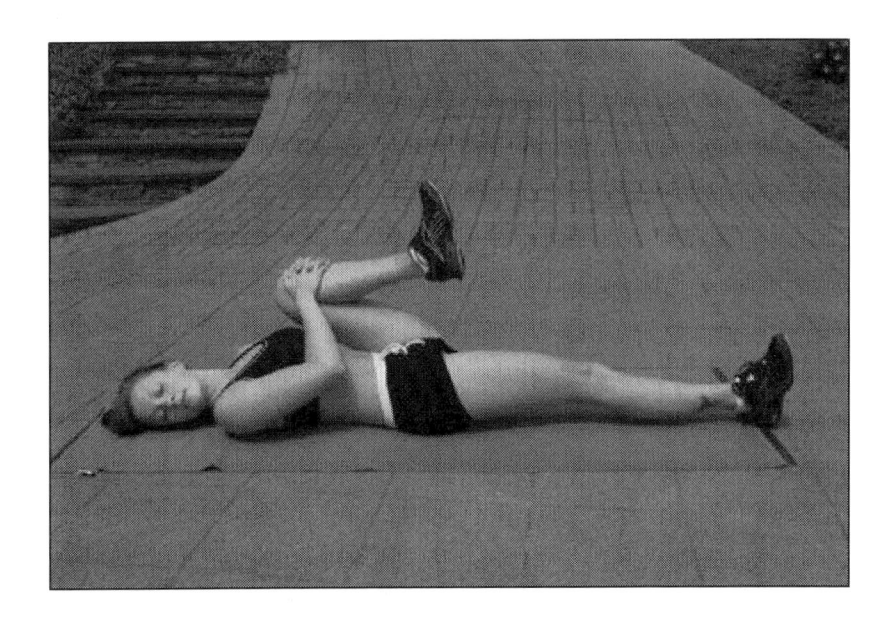

Double Knee To Chest Stretch

For your lower back and legs.

1. Lie flat on your back and then bring up both knees together towards your chest.
2. Wrap your arms over your knees, grabbing the opposite elbow if possible.
3. Curl your head towards your knee.

Hold for 20 to 30 seconds.

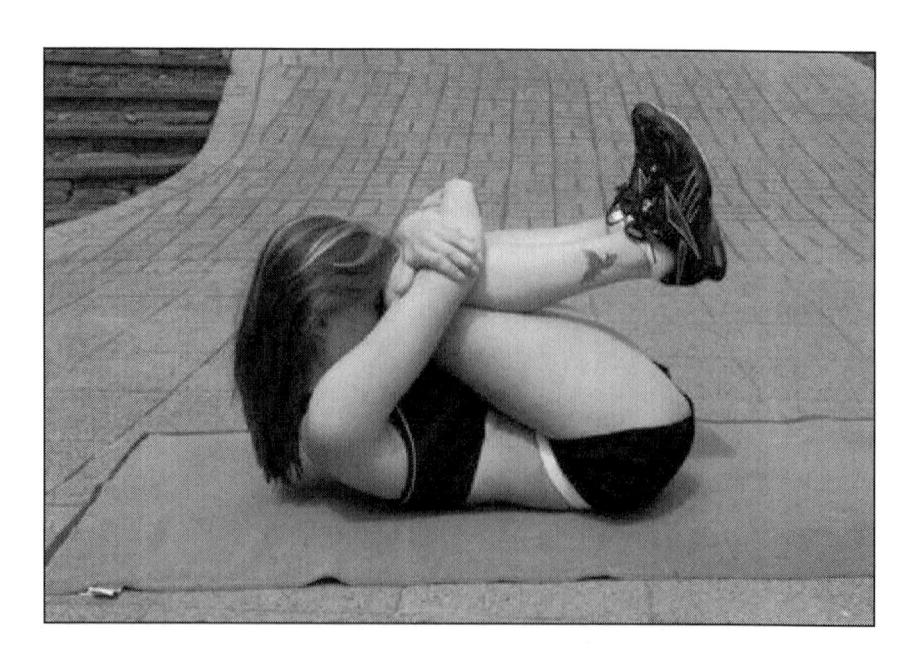

Lower Back And Hip Stretch

1. Lie flat on your back with your arms straight out at a 90 degree angle to your body.
2. Bend your left knee to 90 degrees and pull it gently over your right leg with your right hand.
3. Turn your head so that you are looking at your left hand.

You should feel a gentle stretch in your lower back and hips. Make sure your shoulders are flat on the floor at all times. Hold this stretch for 30 seconds, then repeat on the opposite side.

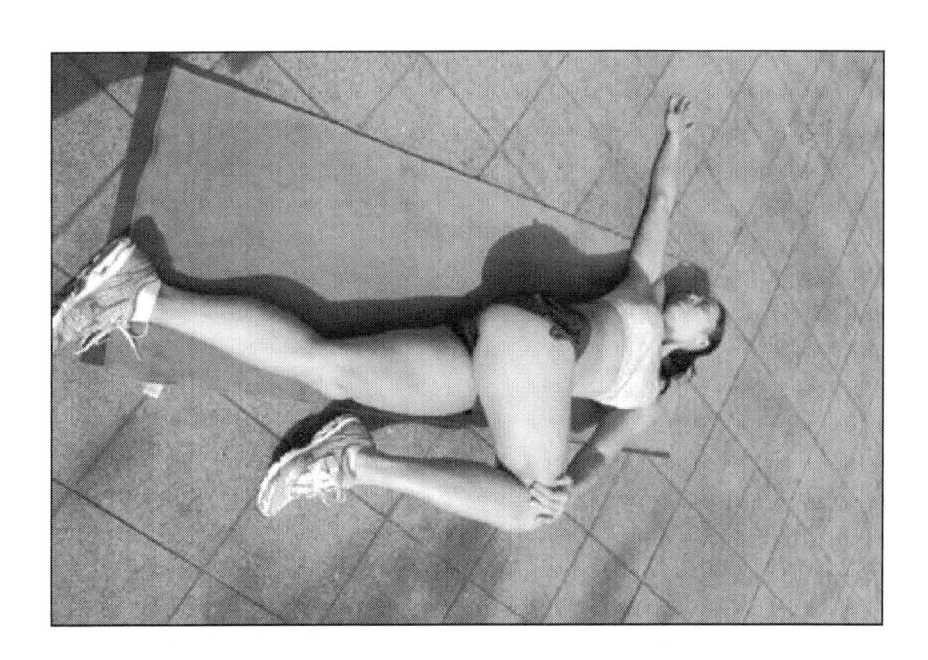

Reaching Upper Back Stretch

1. Stand straight up with your feet shoulder width apart and your arms extended in front of you. Your palms should be facing the floor and your hands crossed.
2. Push your hands forward as far as possible. Keeping your back straight, bend at your hips.
3. Gently lower your head into your arms as you stretch.

You should feel this stretch in your upper back. Focus on reaching forward with your hands and separating your shoulder blades as you do so. Hold this stretch for 10 seconds.

Note: You do not need to lean as far forward as Christine does here. You only need to bend as far as you need to in order to feel the stretch.

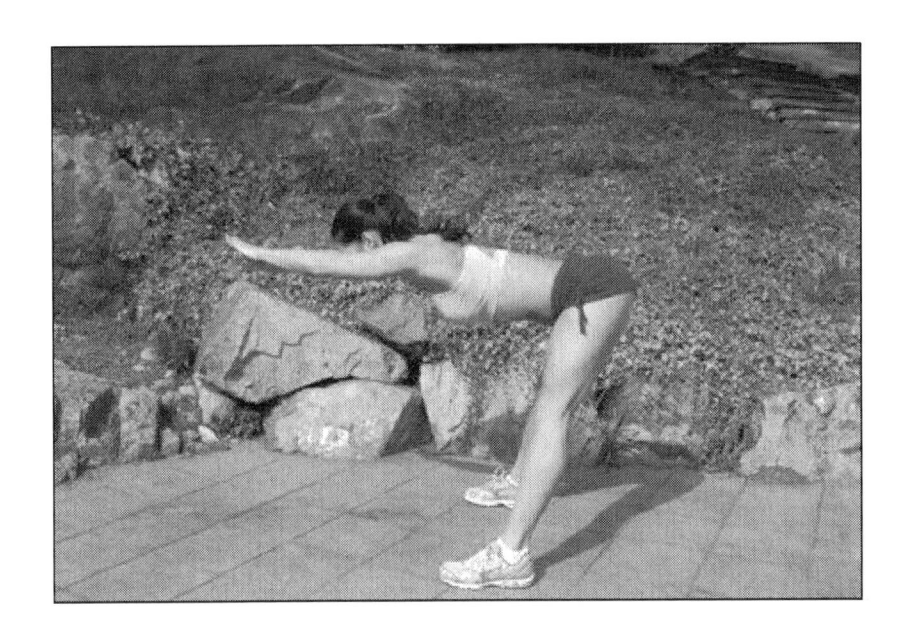

Kneeling Back Arch Stretch

The downward motion works your abs and butt whereas the upward motion stretches your back.

1. Kneel on the floor with your arms and thighs at a 90-degree angle to your body.
2. Look up and allow your back to slump downward. Hold this position for 10 seconds.
3. Let your head slump forward and arch your back upwards. Again hold for 10 seconds.

This stretch should be performed slowly and deliberately. Ensure that your weight is evenly distributed between your knees and hands.

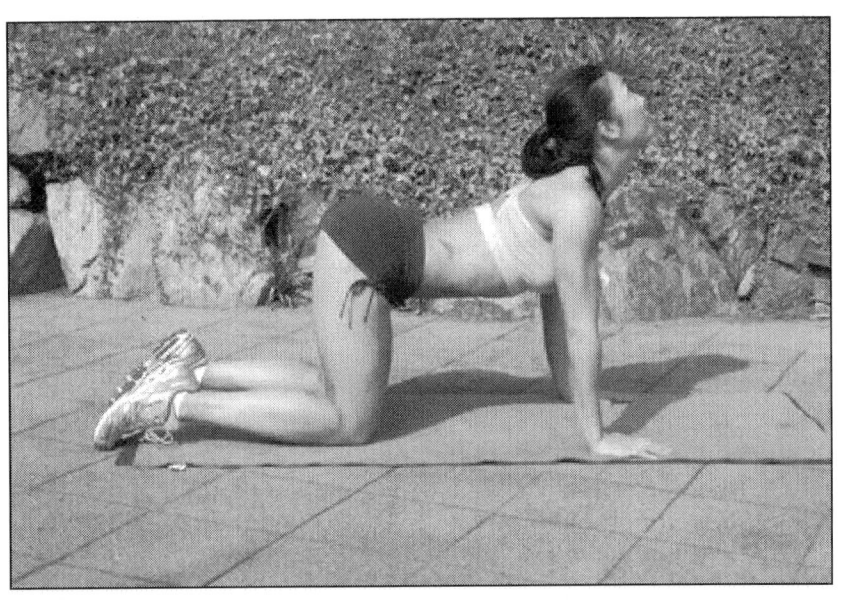

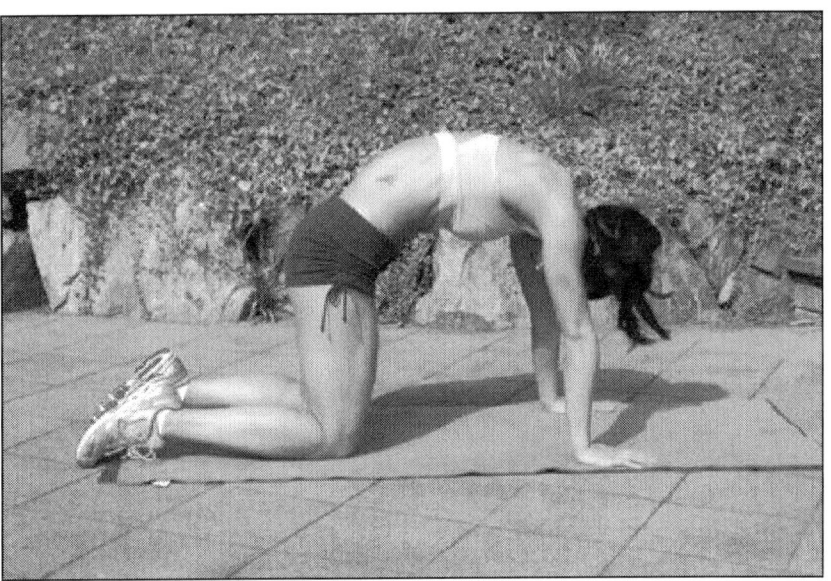

Standing Back Rotation Stretch

This is another great stretch for all of the muscles along your spine.

1. Stand with your feet shoulder width apart and your hands crossed in front of your chest.
2. Slowly rotate your shoulders to one side. Hold for 10 seconds.
3. Repeat in the opposite direction.

If you want to experience a deeper stretch you can use your hands to pull your shoulders, and therefore your body, further around.

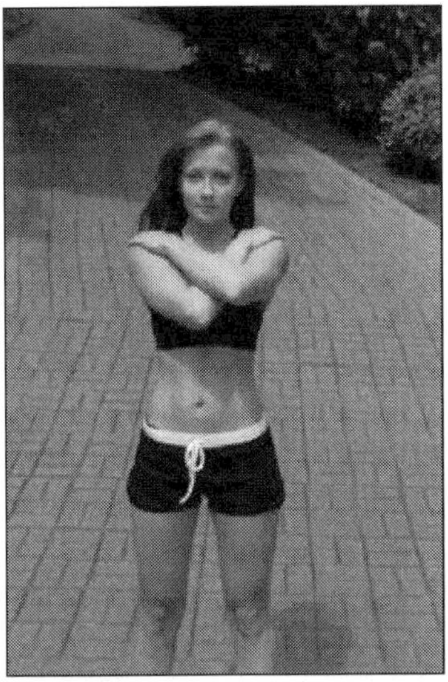

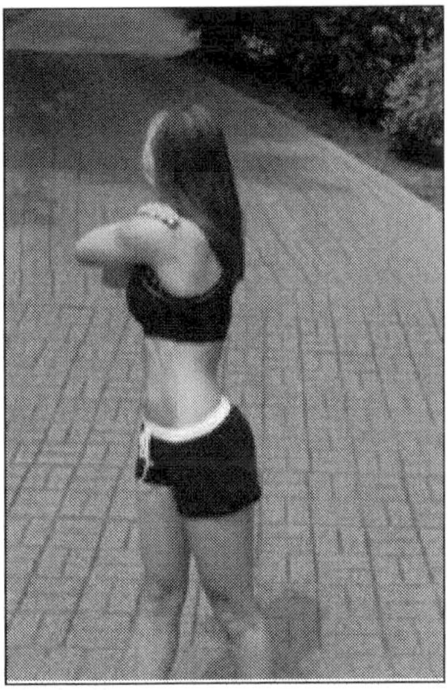

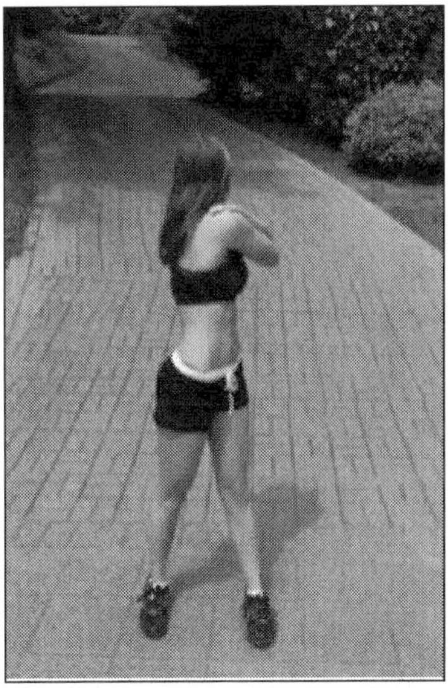

Spinal Twist

1. Sit on the floor with your right leg out straight.
2. Bend your left leg and cross it over your right leg. Place the left foot on the outside of your right knee.
3. Bend your right elbow and rest it on the outside of your upper left thigh. Keep your left arm on the floor for support.
4. Slowly turn your head to look over your left shoulder while rotating your upper body.

You should feel this stretch in your lower back and hip. Do not hold your breath while performing this stretch. Breathe easily and naturally.

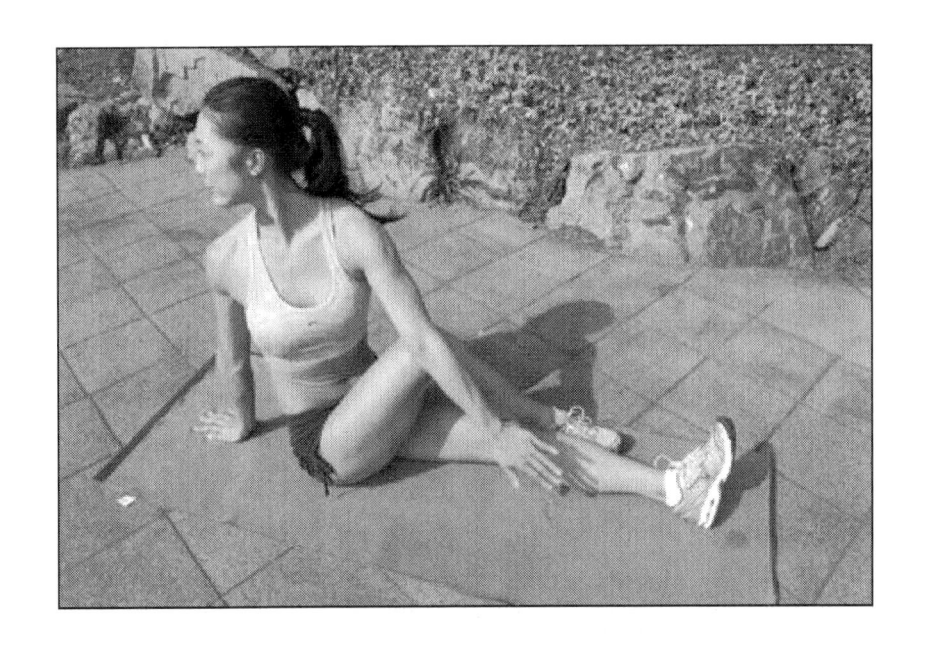

Squat Stretch

1. Begin by standing with your heels a comfortable distance apart (at least 12 inches) and your toes pointed out at roughly a 15-degree angle.
2. Squat down so that your knees are to the outside of your shoulders and your knees are directly above your big toes.
3. Hold for 30 seconds.

The squat stretch will work your lower legs, knees, back, ankles, Achilles tendons and groin.

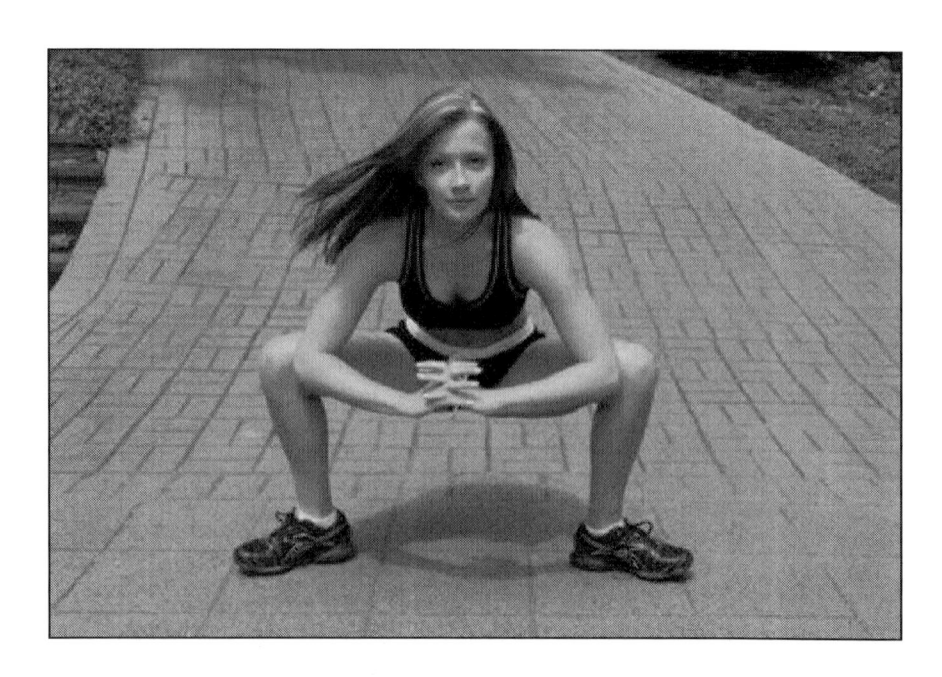

Cobra Stretch

1. Begin lying on the ground with your heels together. Your eyes should be looking forward, not at the ground.
2. Place your palms on the ground underneath your shoulders.
3. Straighten your arms and look up. This will raise your stomach off the ground. Keep your hips on the ground.

This exercise will stretch your stomach and relieve tension from your back. Take it easy when first performing this stretch as most people are not used to back bending.

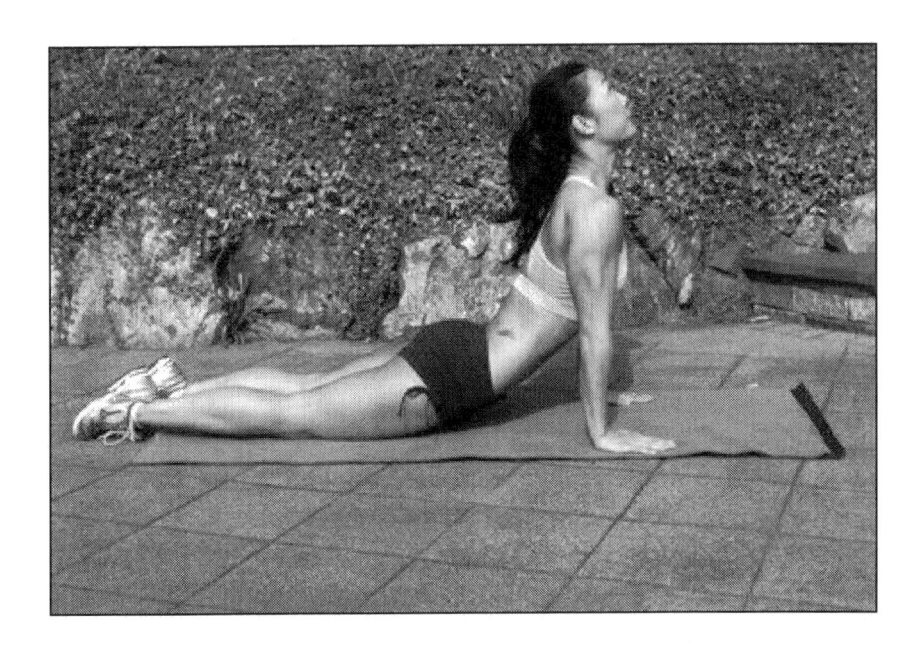

Hamstring Stretch

This will stretch your hamstrings, and your lower back as well.

1. Sitting on the ground, straighten your left leg in front of you. Although it will be straight it should not be rigidly locked.
2. Bend your right leg so the sole of your right foot is against your left thigh.
3. Bend forward from your hips, looking forward at all times and keeping your back straight. You should feel a slight stretch in the hamstrings (back of your right upper leg) and perhaps on the left side of your lower back.
4. Do an easy stretch for 30 seconds.
5. Repeat for the opposite leg.

Never rush your stretches. Take your time, take slow, calming breathes, and THINK your muscles into a relaxed state. The foot of the outstretched leg should never turns outwards as this will lead to a misalignment in your hips. If you are not very flexible or a beginner you can wrap a towel around your feet to aid in the stretch. Always remember to never force the stretch to the point of pain.

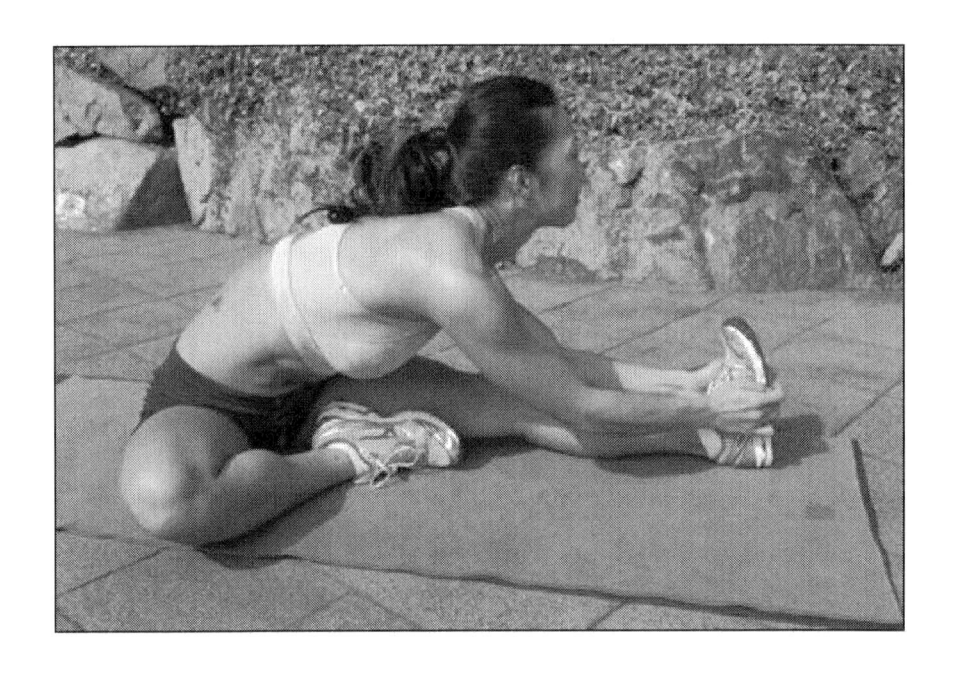

Lying Groin Stretch

1. Lie down on the ground with your hands on your chest and the soles of your feet together.
2. Let your knees fall apart and let gravity alone pull your knees down. You should feel a gentle stretch in your groin area.
3. Hold this position for 40 seconds, breathing slowly and calmly at all times.

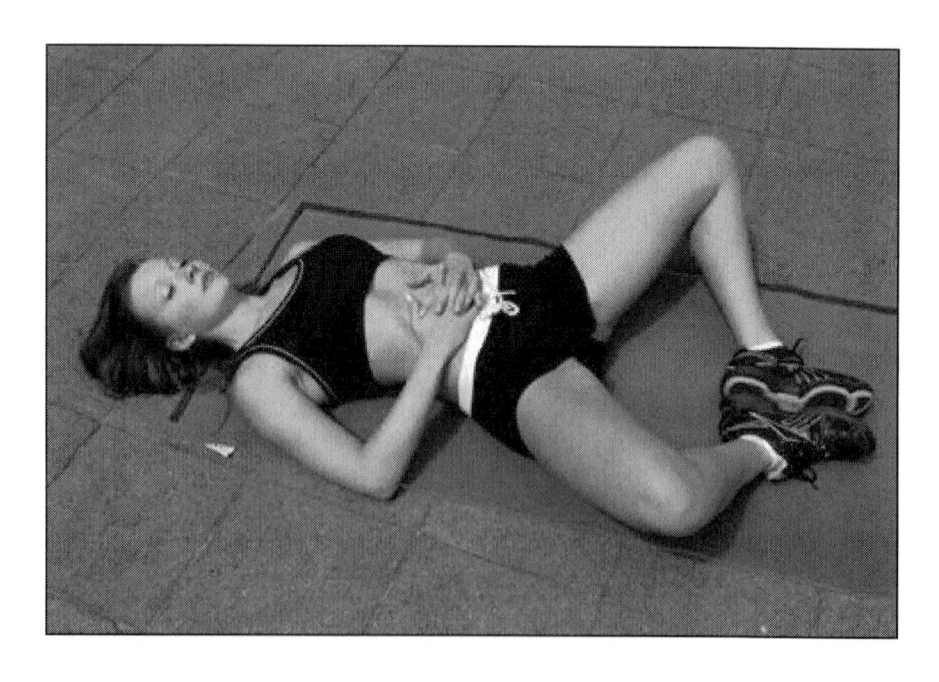

Neck Stretch

This stretch works your upper spine and neck while also helping to reduce tension in those areas.

1. Lie flat on the floor with your knees bent. Interlace your fingers behind your head above the ear level.
2. Lift your head with your hands, gently curling your neck and upper spine upwards.

This stretch can be held for 5 to 10 seconds. Repeat 3 to 4 times.

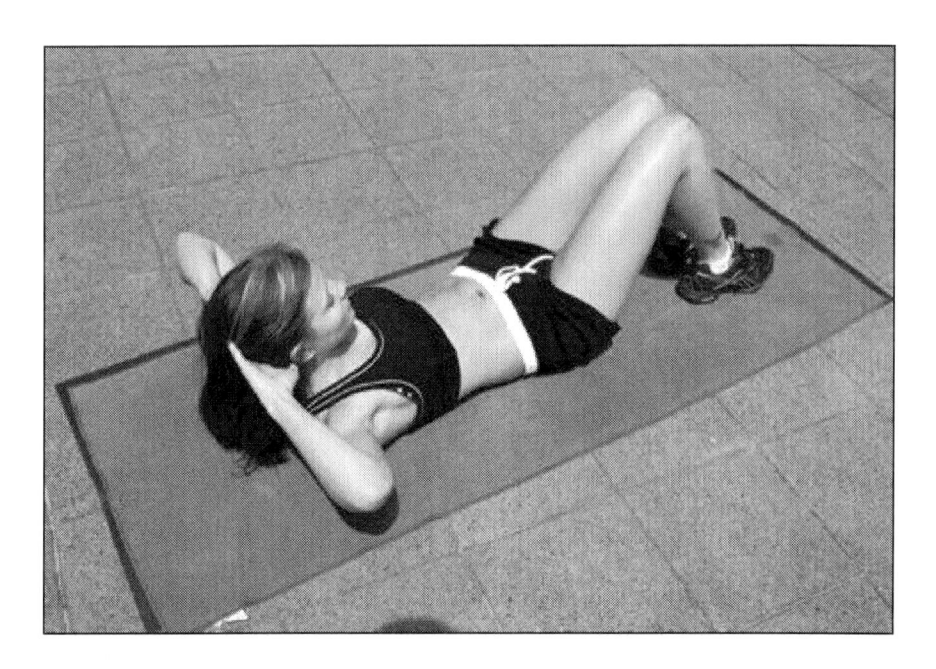

4 Point Neck Stretch

1. Bend your head forward so that your chin touches your upper chest.
2. Bend your head backwards so that you are looking at the ceiling.
3. Bend your head to the left and right side.

Hold each position for 5 to 10 seconds.

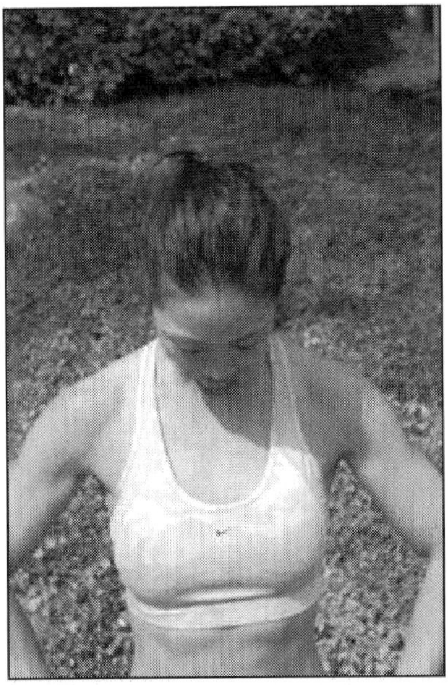
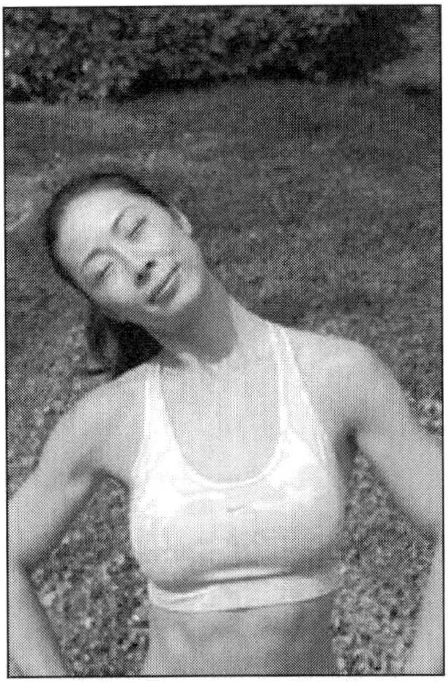
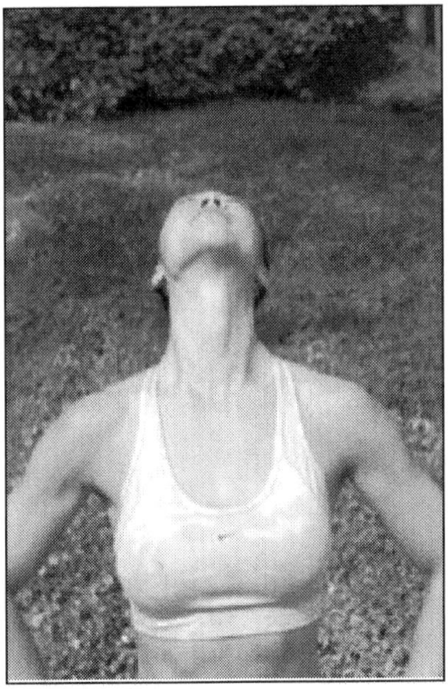
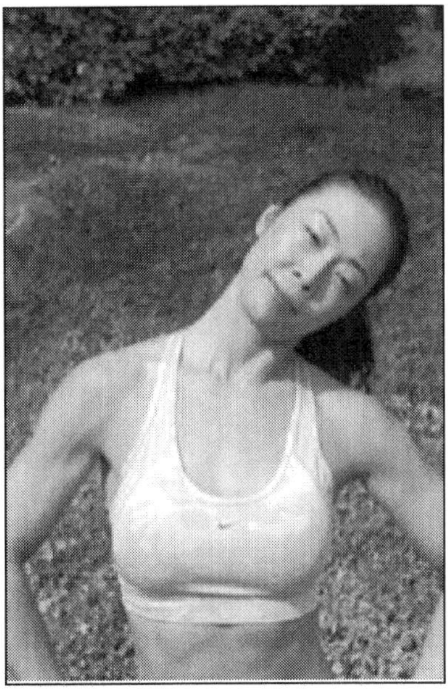

"Praying" Stretch

1. Kneel down on the floor with your knees separated.
2. Reach forward as far as you can with both arms and grab the mat or carpet if you can.
3. Pull backwards with straight arms and back while keeping your palms pressed down.
4. Hold for 15 seconds.

You should feel this stretch in your arms, shoulders and upper back. You can also do this stretch with one arm at a time for great control, if you wish.

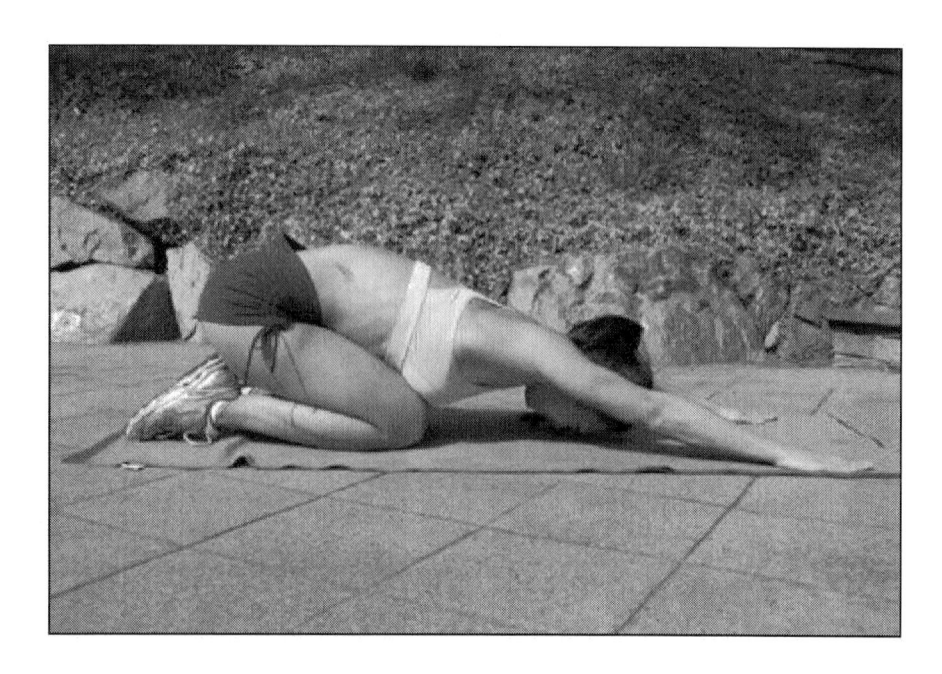

Cross Shoulder Stretch

1. Place your right hand by your left shoulder.
2. Use your left hand to pull your right elbow across your chest.
3. Hold this stretch for 15 seconds.

You should feel this stretch in your shoulder and upper back.

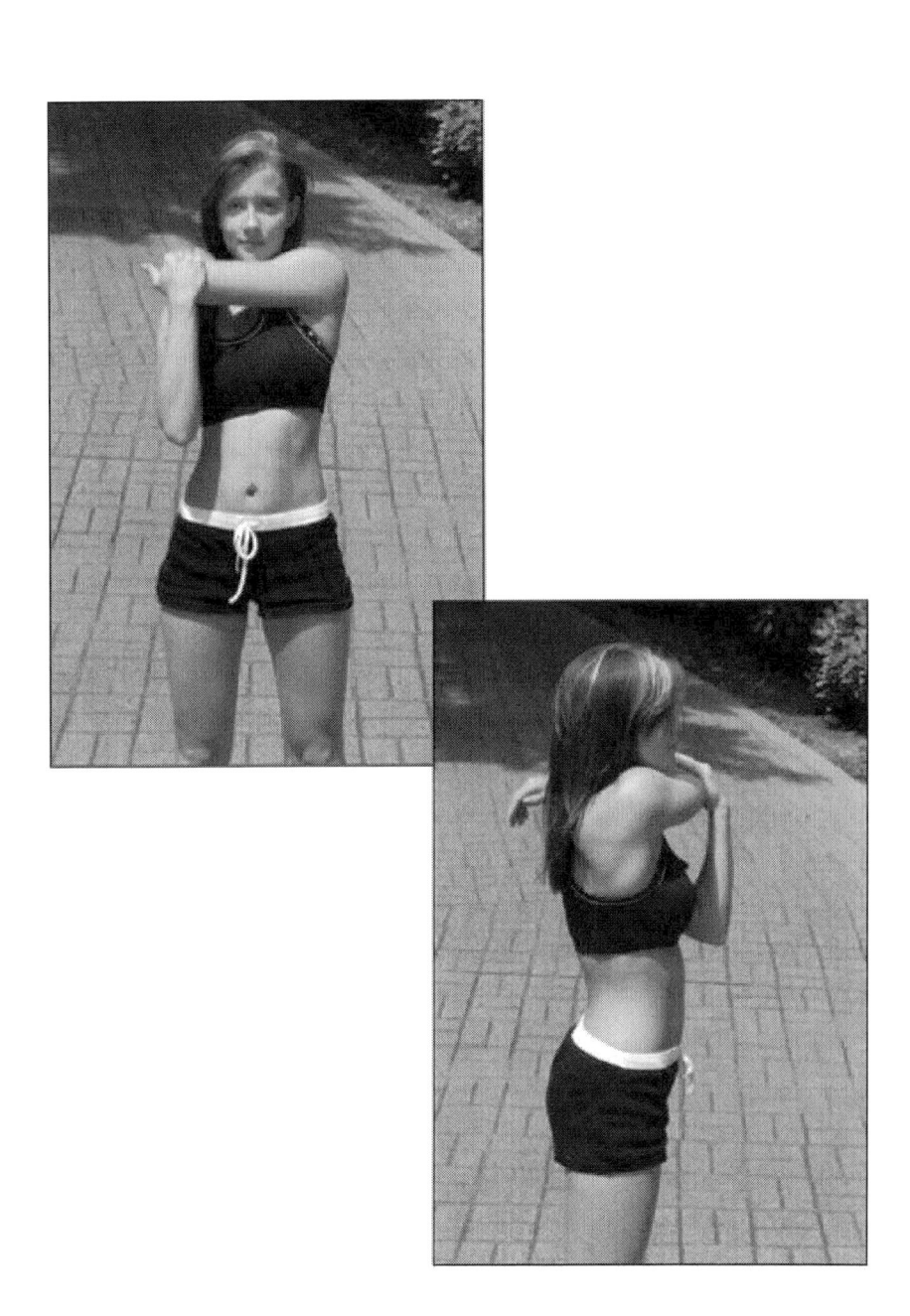

Back Shoulder Stretch

1. With your left elbow in the air, reach behind your back with your left hand.
2. With your right elbow towards the floor, reach up with your right hand, palm out, and grab your left hand with your fingers.
3. Hold this stretch for 15 seconds.

If you are not flexible enough for your hands to meet behind your back make up the distance by using a towel. As you gain in flexibility inch up the towel, bringing your hands closer together, until you no longer need it.

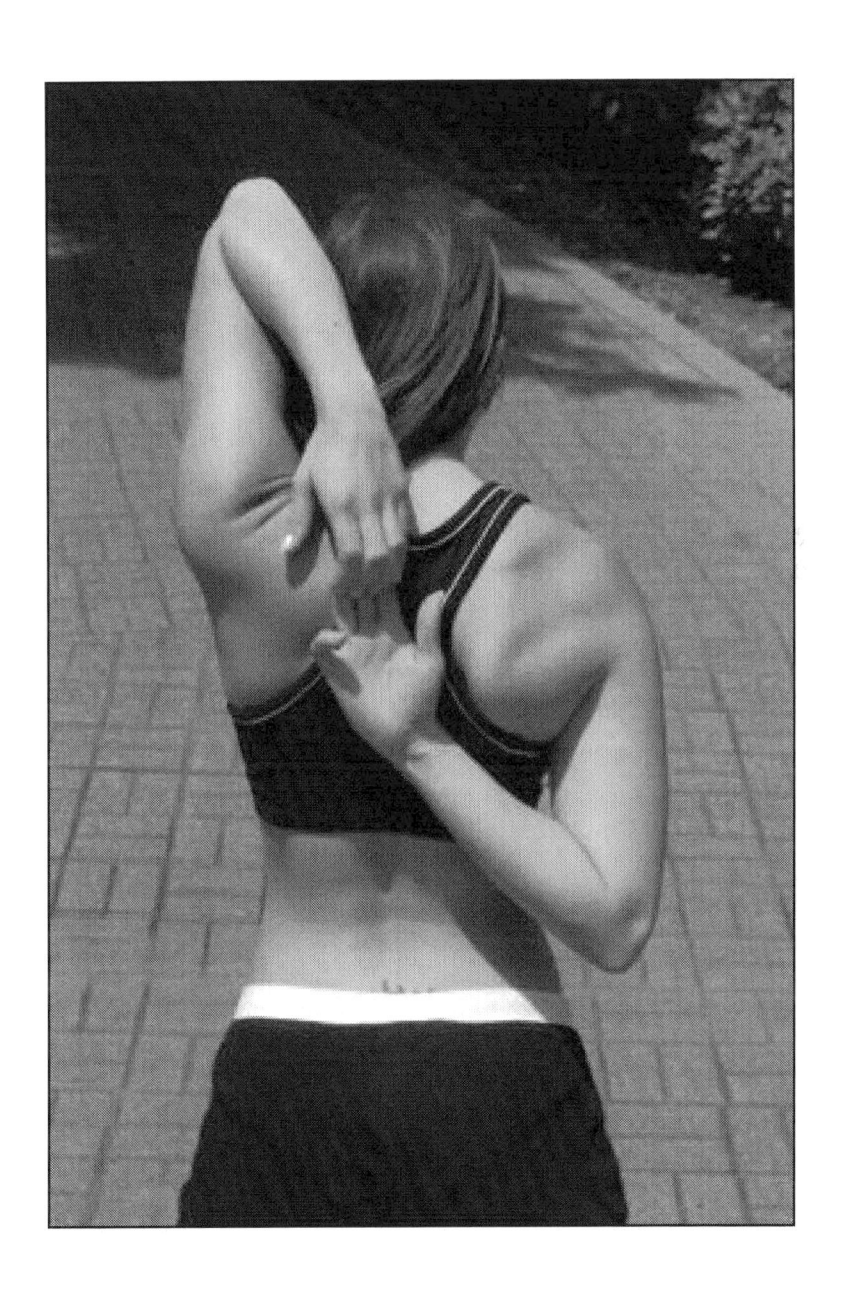

Straight Arm Stretch

1. Interlace your fingers in front of you and extend your arms with the palms out.
2. Hold this stretch for 15 seconds.
3. Relax, then raise your hands above your head. Extend your arms again and hold for another 15 seconds.

You should feel a stretch in your shoulders, upper back, hands, fingers, forearms and wrists.

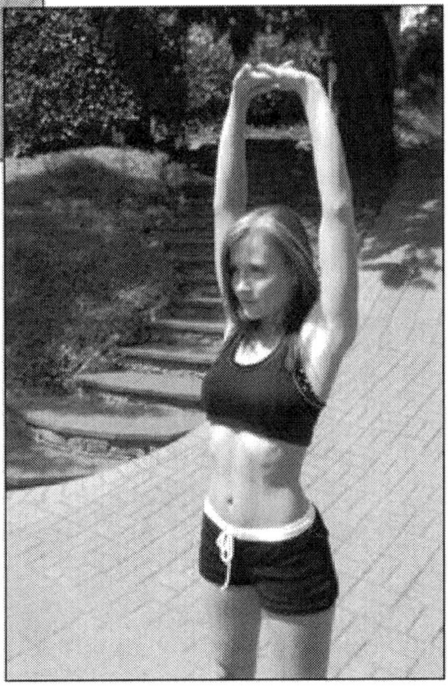

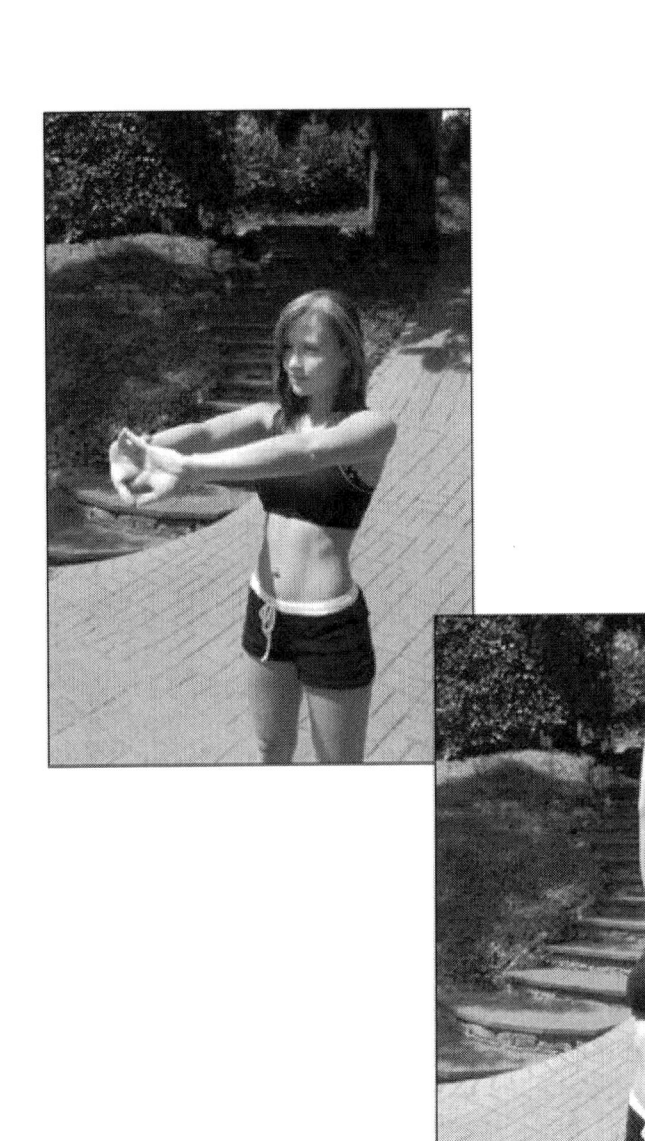

Straight Arm Behind Back Stretch

1. Interlace your fingers with the palms up behind your back.
2. Straighten your arms while turning your elbows inward.
3. If you are able, lift your arms up and hold an easy stretch for 10 - 15 seconds.

You should feel this stretch in your arms, shoulders and chest.

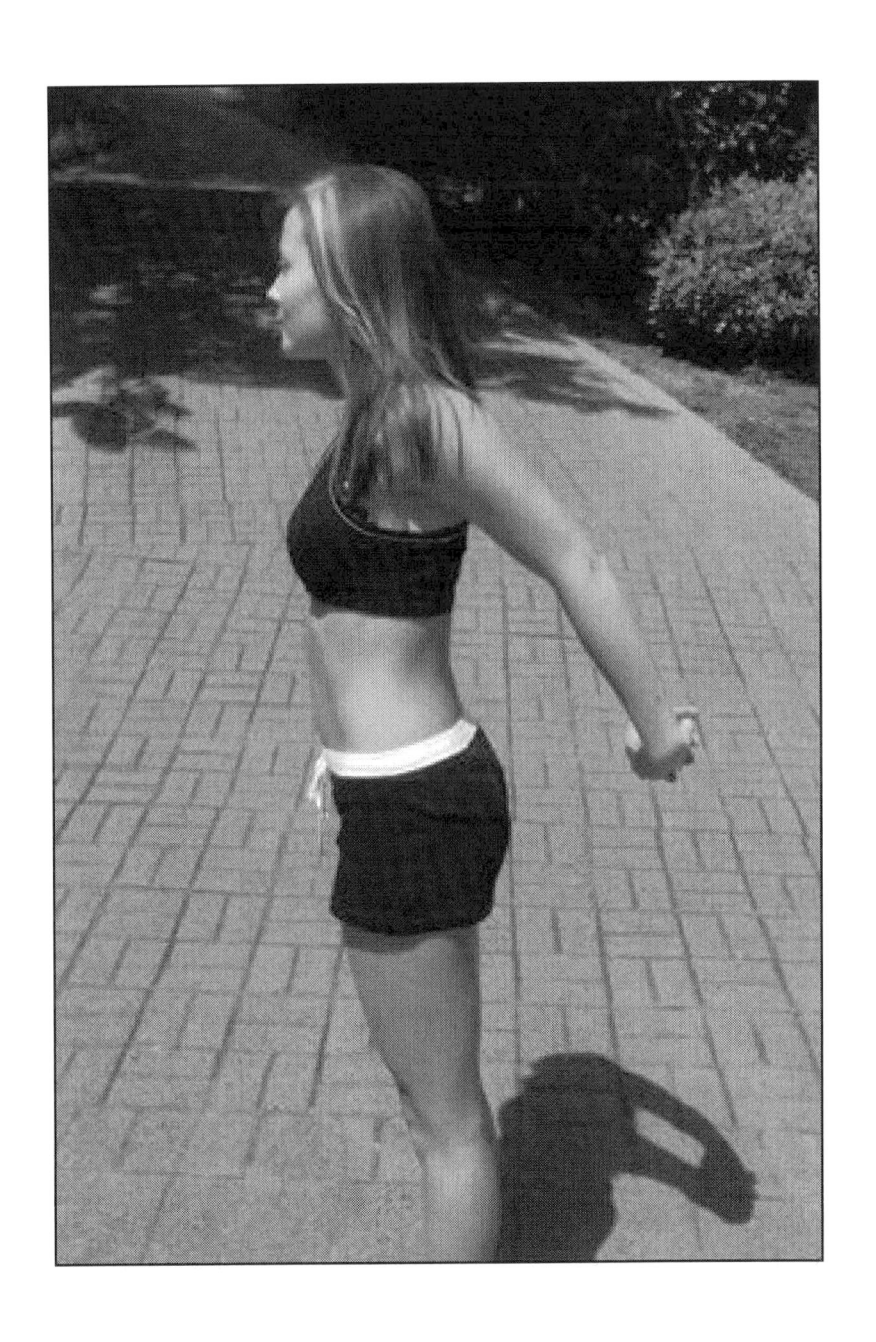

Cross Over Shoulder Stretch

1. Stand with your knees bent while crossing your arms and grabbing the back of your legs just above the knees.
2. Start to raise your shoulders upwards until you feel a stretch in your upper back and shoulders.

Avoid twisting or turning to one side while performing this stretch.

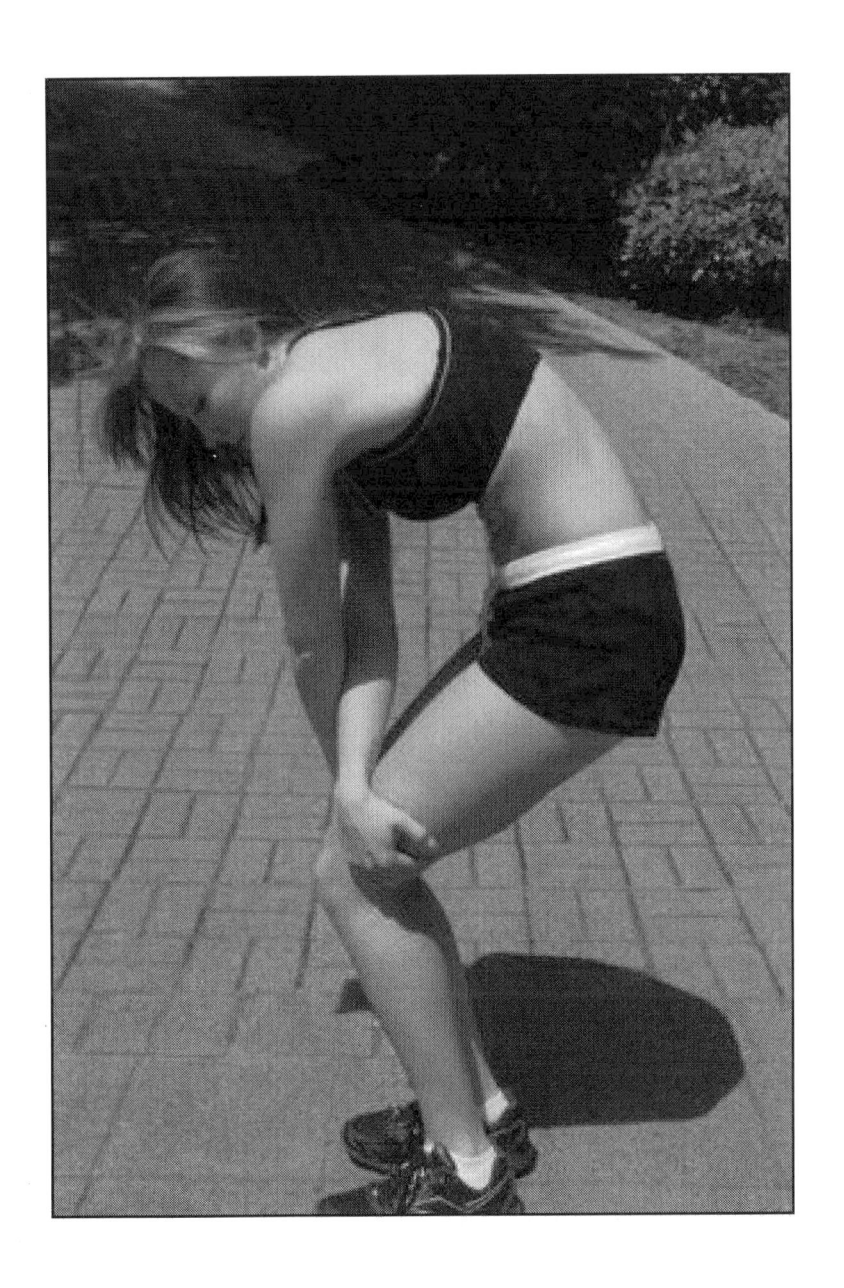

Standing Waist Stretch

1. Stand straight up with your feet shoulder width apart and your toes pointed forward.
2. Place one hand on your hip as you raise the opposite arm above your head.
3. Keeping your knees slightly bent slowly bend at the waist towards the side with your hands on your hip.
4. Move slowly - stopping when you feel a good stretch on the side of your body. Hold a gentle stretch for 10 to 15 seconds.

This stretch will also build strength along the side of your body as well.

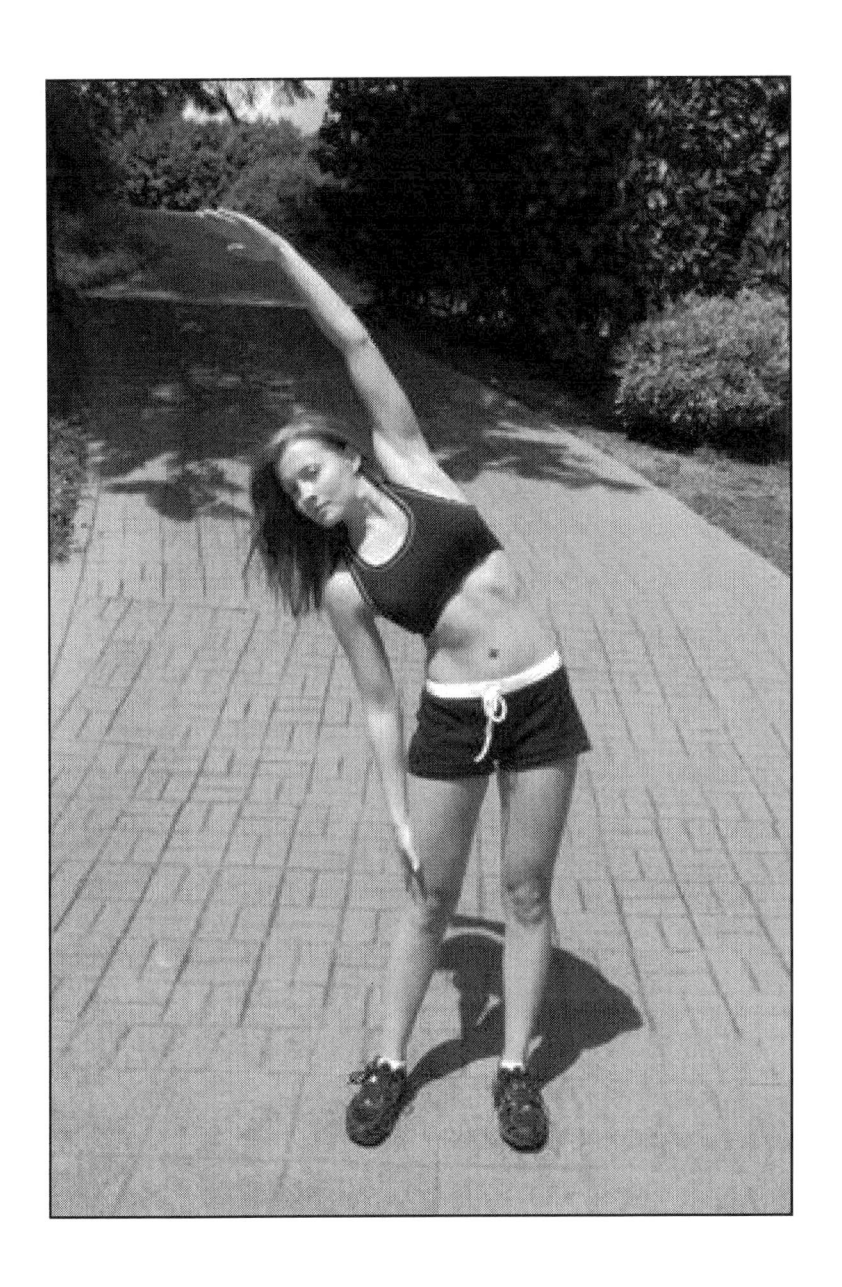

Bent-Over Upper Back Stretch

1. Place both hands face down on a surface such as a fence, ledge or mantel that is roughly as high as your hips.
2. Bending at the waist let your body drop down while keeping your knees slightly bent.
3. Hold this gentle stretch for 30 seconds.

This will really stretch your upper back and shoulders as well as your chest. As your get better at it you will really feel a nice stretch in your spine as well.

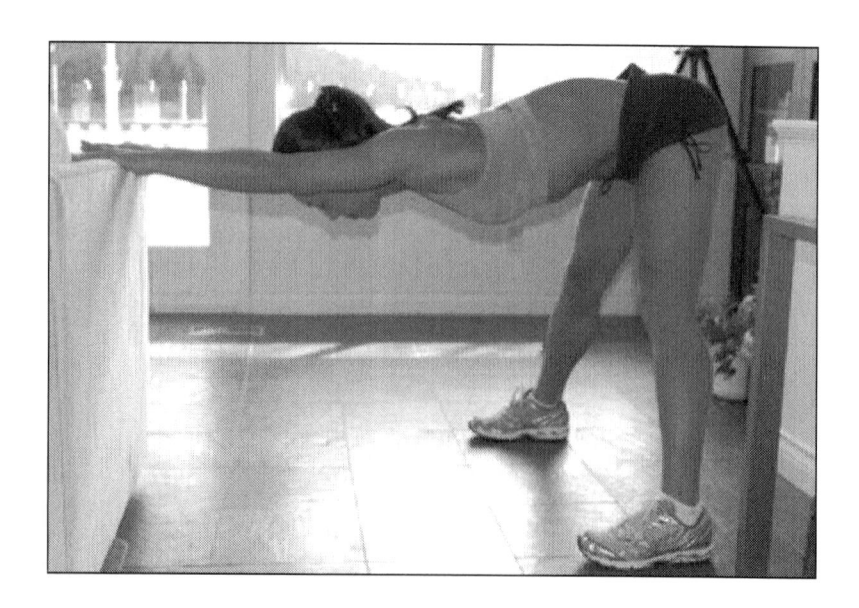

Table Maker Stretch

1. Begin sitting on the ground with your legs straight out in front of you and your palms on the ground fingers pointed forward.
2. Lift your butt and bend your knees while you simultaneously bend your head backwards to look at the ceiling. You are trying to make your thighs, stomach and chest as flat as possible forming a "table".
3. Hold for a second then bring your butt down again so that it slides between your arms. You should be back in the starting position again.
4. Repeat 10 times.

Additional Notes

- This is a variation of the table maker. The only difference between it and this stretch is that you hold the table maker for time.
- This is a great stretch for your shoulders and spine.
- Primary areas worked - shoulders, back (lower, mid, upper), hips

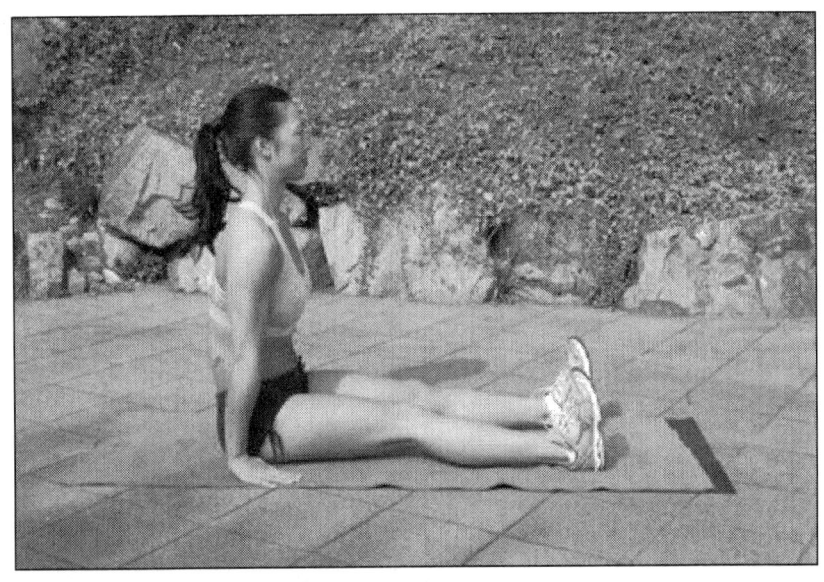

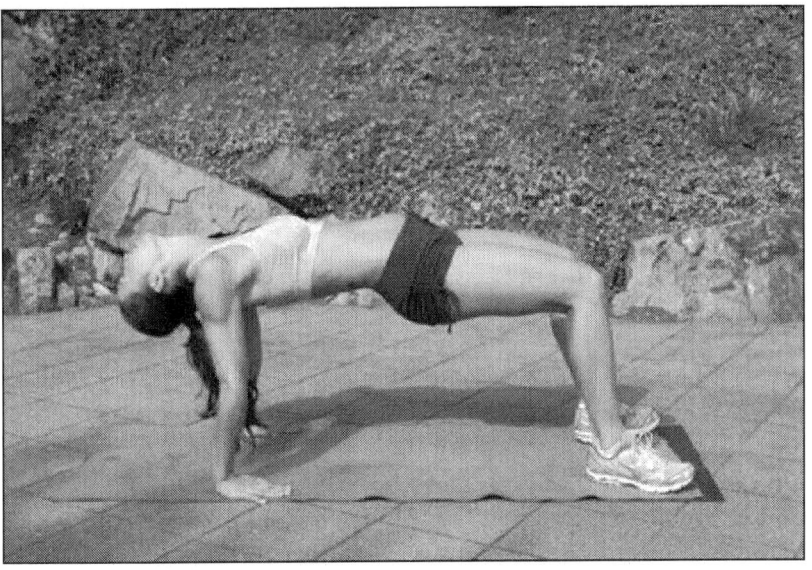

Dynamic Bridging Stretch

1. Begin lying on your back with your feet tucked in behind your butt. Your hands should be palms down beside your head with the fingers pointed backwards.
2. Raise your butt off the floor while you arch your back backwards. As you do so you will roll onto your head towards your forehead and nose.
3. Press back with your feet forcing your nose towards the floor. Hold for a second then relax so that your nose comes off the floor.
4. Repeat this gentle back and forth motion 10 times.

Additional Notes

- This stretch builds strength and flexibility throughout your entire body, including your abdominals, hips, buttocks, legs and shoulders. It is especially beneficial for your neck and spine, however.
- Take it easy when performing this stretch. If you can't touch your nose to the floor or even your forehead don't worry about it. Just do the best you can.
- Primary areas worked - back (lower, mid, upper), neck

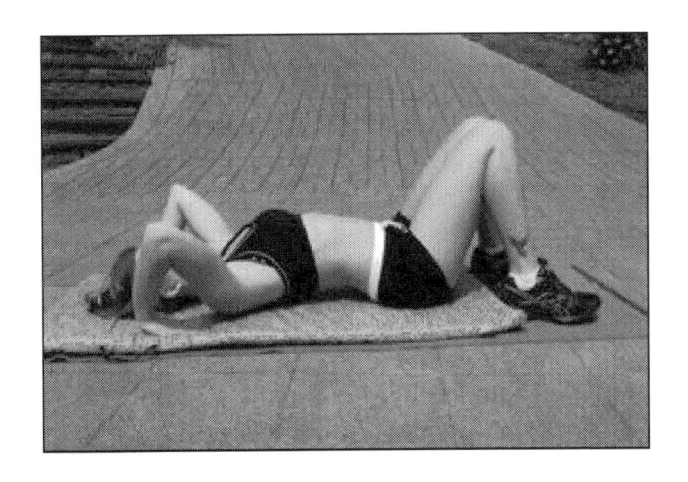

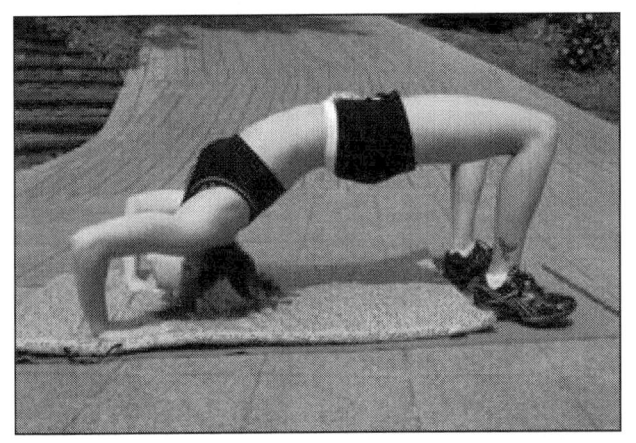

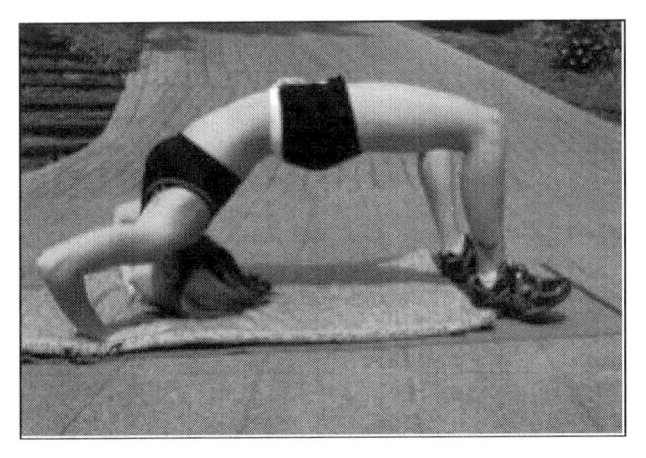

Back Strengthening Exercises

Grounded Back Twist

1. Take a wide stance, double shoulder length at minimum.
2. Bend your knees while keeping your back straight and place the palms of your hands on the inside of your knees. Use your hands to gently push your knees further out laterally.
3. Turn your head so that you are looking over your right shoulder. Twist your upper body at the same time as if you are trying to look at the wall behind you.
4. Hold for 5 seconds then repeat on the opposite side.
5. Repeat this 5 times.

Additional Notes

- This will stretch your lower back and will also help ground your energy. You will feel a greater sense of calm and focus when you have finished this exercise.
- Breathe in through your nose as you look over you shoulder. Exhale when you look forward.
- Primary areas worked - lower back

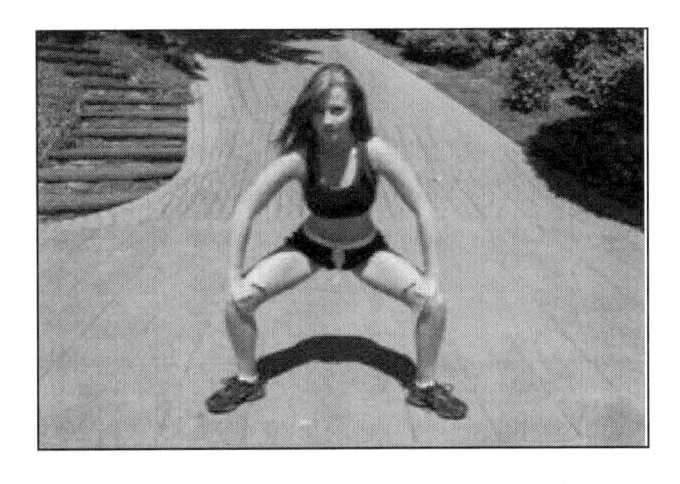

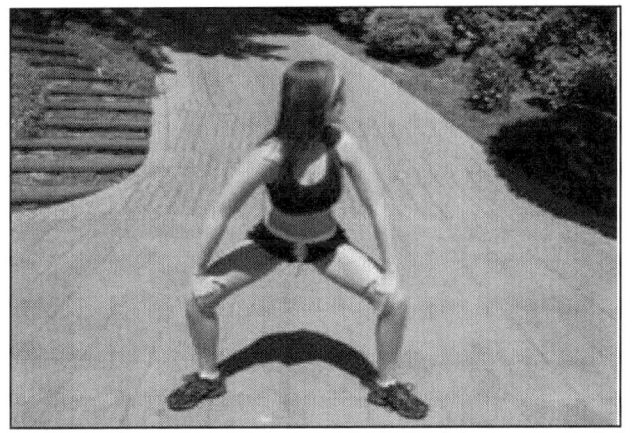

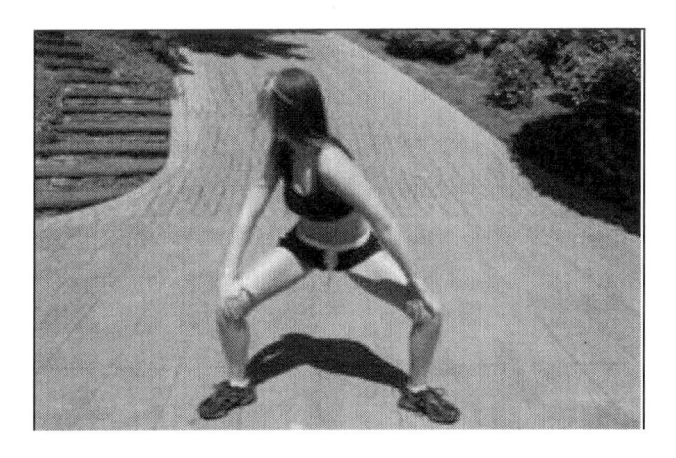

Sumo Squat Stretch

1. Begin with your heels slightly wider than shoulder width apart and your toes turned out to either side almost like a clown.
2. Keeping your back straight bend your knees and lower your body as far as you can. Breathe in through your nose as you do so. You should feel a gentle stretch in your hips, groin and lower back.
3. Breathe in through your nose as you raise your body back to the starting position.
4. Repeat this motion 5 to 10 times depending on how you're feeling.

Additional Points

- Turn out your toes as far as you can while still maintaining your balance. If your legs are really stiff simply turn them out as far as you can.
- When you lower your body always look straight ahead. This will help keep your back straight.
- Primary areas worked - lower back, hip, groin

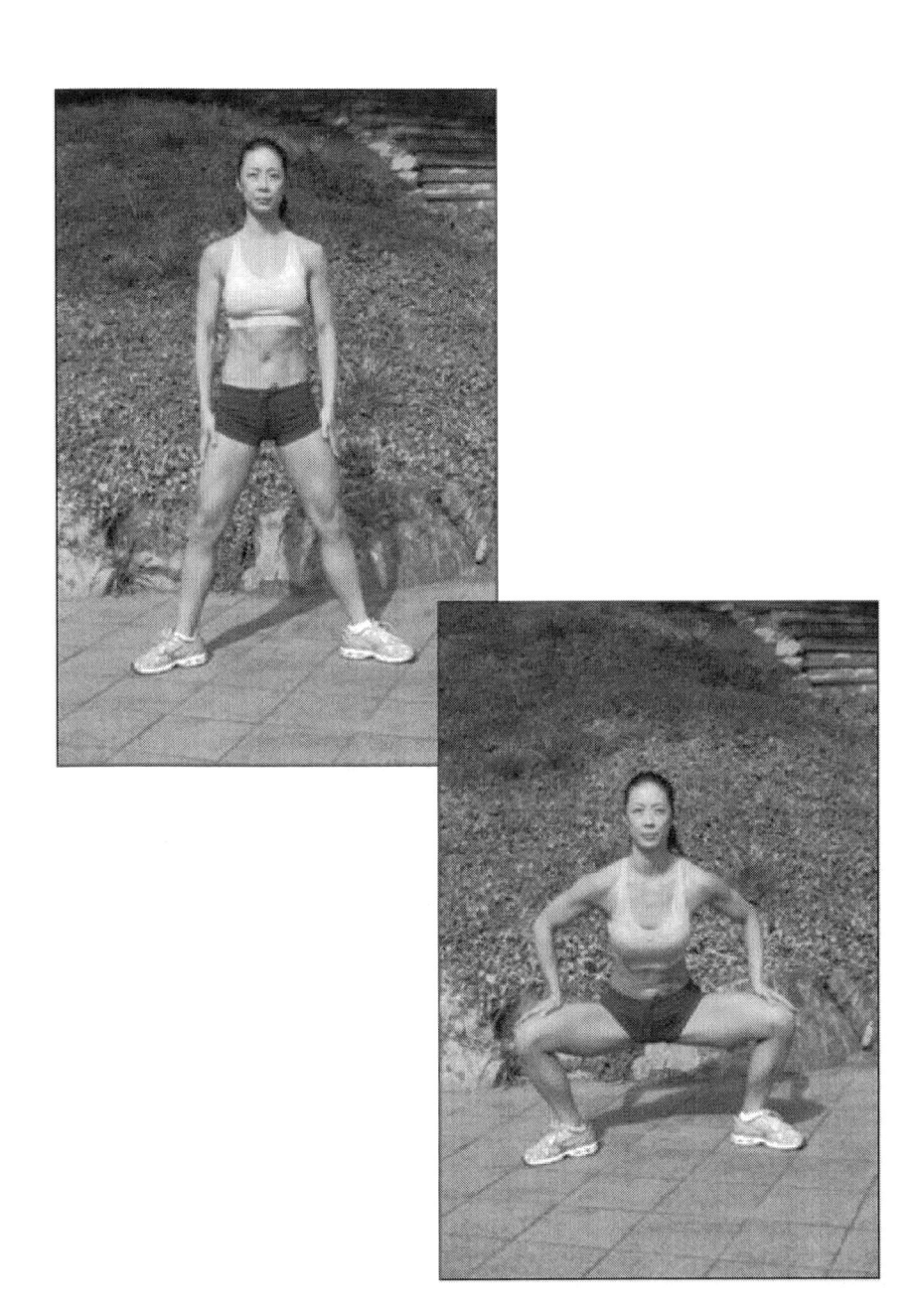

Sumo Squat Kicks

1. Begin in the Sumo Squat Position with your back straight and your toes out.
2. Squat down keeping your back straight while always looking forward.
3. Balance on your right foot while you bring your left foot towards it.
4. Lightly touch your left heal to your right foot and then kick your left foot to the side so that it touches your left hand.
5. Bring your left foot back to the Sumo Squat Position then repeat on the opposite side.
6. Repeat 10 times or until you feel loose.

Additional Points

- This exercise will increase flexibility and strength in your back and thighs while improving your balance.
- If you can't touch your hand to your foot when you kick up don't worry about it. Simply touch the palm of your hand to your leg. Just do the best you can.
- In Japan Sumo wrestlers do hundreds of these movements in a day. If a 500-pound man can do them you really don't have an excuse, do you? ;)
- Primary areas worked - lower back, hip, groin, quadriceps

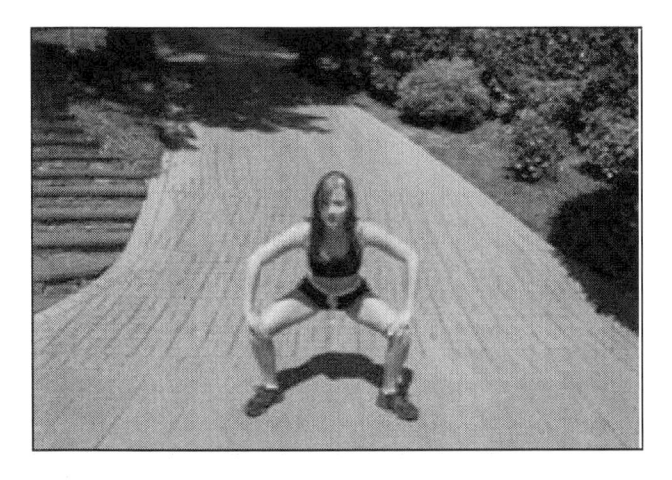

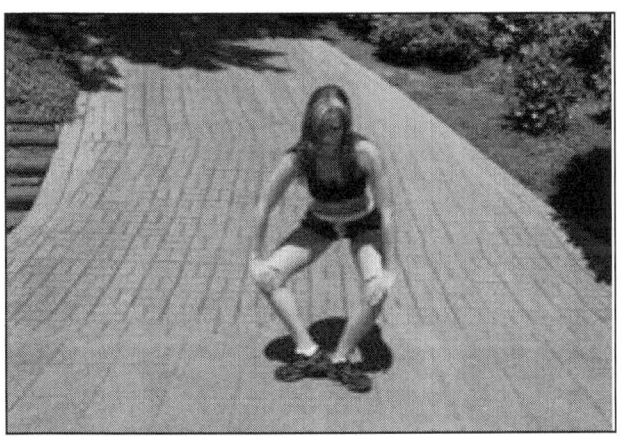

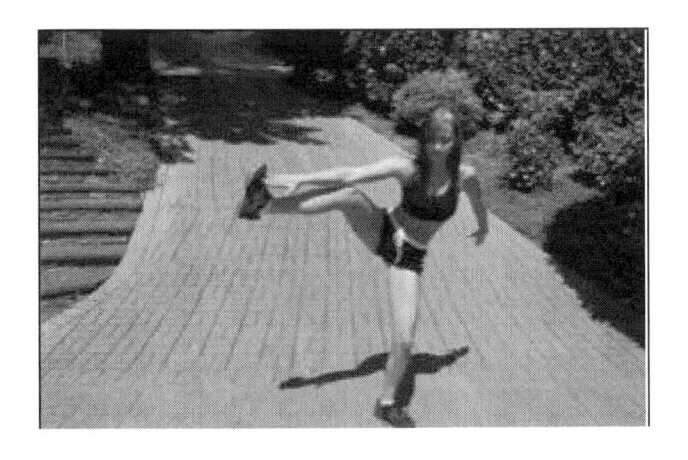

Ying/Yang Bends

1. Begin standing with your feet shoulder width apart and your knees slightly bend. Place your hands on the back of your hips / lower back for support.
2. Look up at the ceiling and breathe in through your nose as you bend your back backwards. Go as far as you can while maintaining your balance. Imagine that you are trying to look at the wall behind you.
3. Bend forward at the waist while exhaling your breath through your nose. Touch your hands to the floor. If you have trouble reaching the floor it is OK to bend your knees more.
4. Repeat this motion 10 times.

Additional Notes

- Remember to go slowly and deliberately. Don't rush anything.
- Keep your knees slightly bent at all times. This takes pressure off the lower back.
- This exercise is great for the lower back, spine and waist.
- Primary areas worked - lower back, abdominals

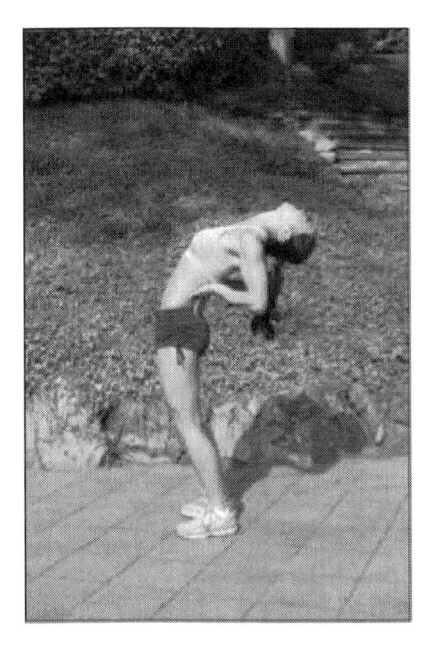

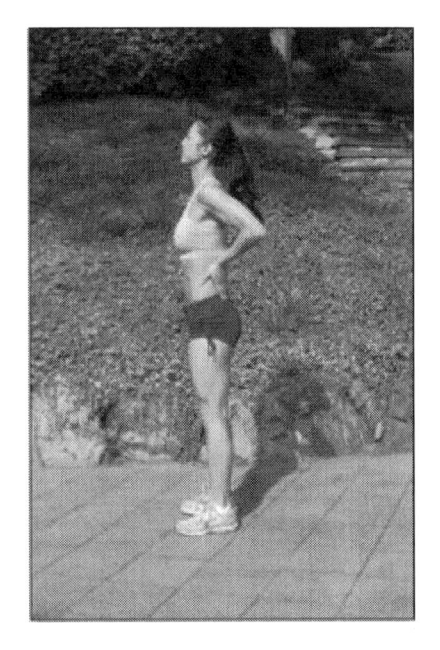

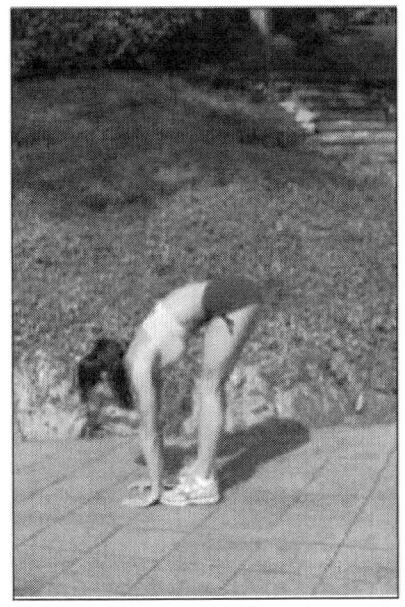

Tai Chi Waist Turner

1. Stand straight up with your knees slightly bent and your feet shoulder width apart. Your arms should be hanging loosely by your sides.
2. Turn your head and body to one side, then twist your body to the opposite. Move fast enough so that you generate the centrifugal force necessary to swing your arms. At the end of each twist your hands should gently slap your lower back and kidneys.
3. Do 50 to 100 reps.

Additional Notes

- This movement will loosen up your waist while massaging your internal organs and re-aligning your spine.
- You should never consciously move your arms. The only thing moving them should be the force generated by the twisting motion.
- The slapping of your arms and hands against your body is what generates the massage and is very beneficial for your internal organs.
- Primary areas worked - lower back

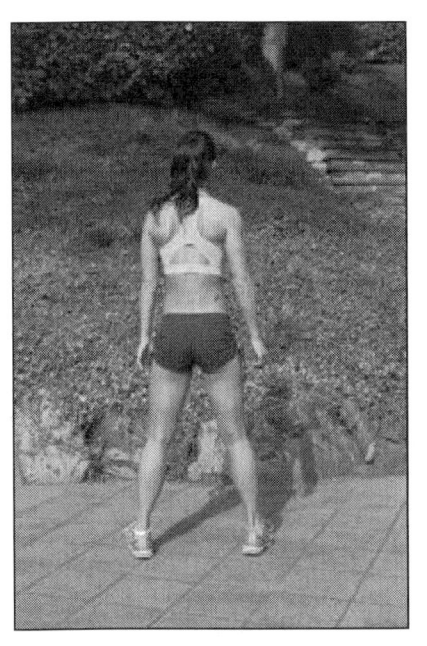

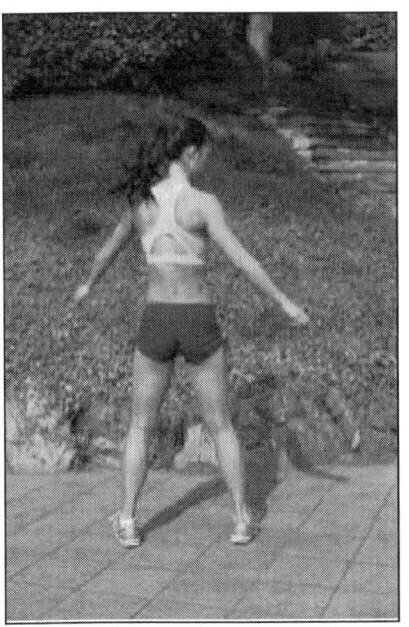

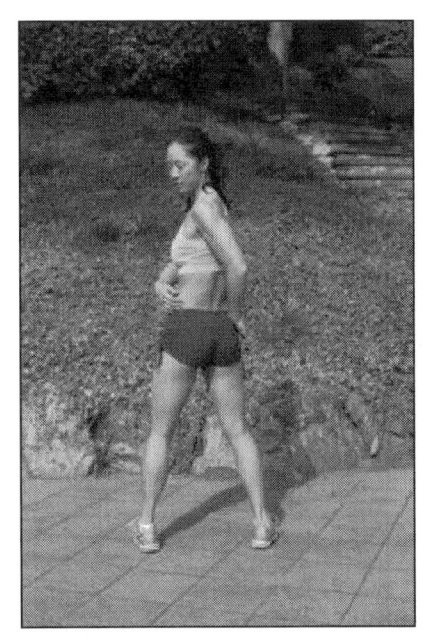

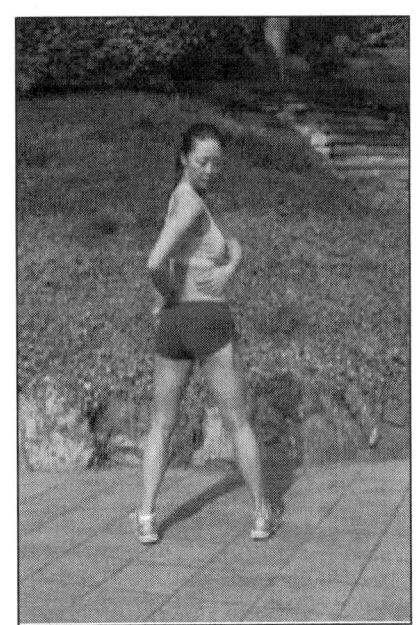

Gymnastic Shoulder Shrugs

1. Begin standing with your feet shoulder width apart.
2. Raise your hands above your head with your palms pointed down.
3. Shrug your shoulders up, hold for a second or two, and then relax.
4. Do 10 to 15 reps.

Additional Notes

- When you bring your hands above your head imagine that you are holding onto a large beach ball.
- Primary areas worked - upper back

73

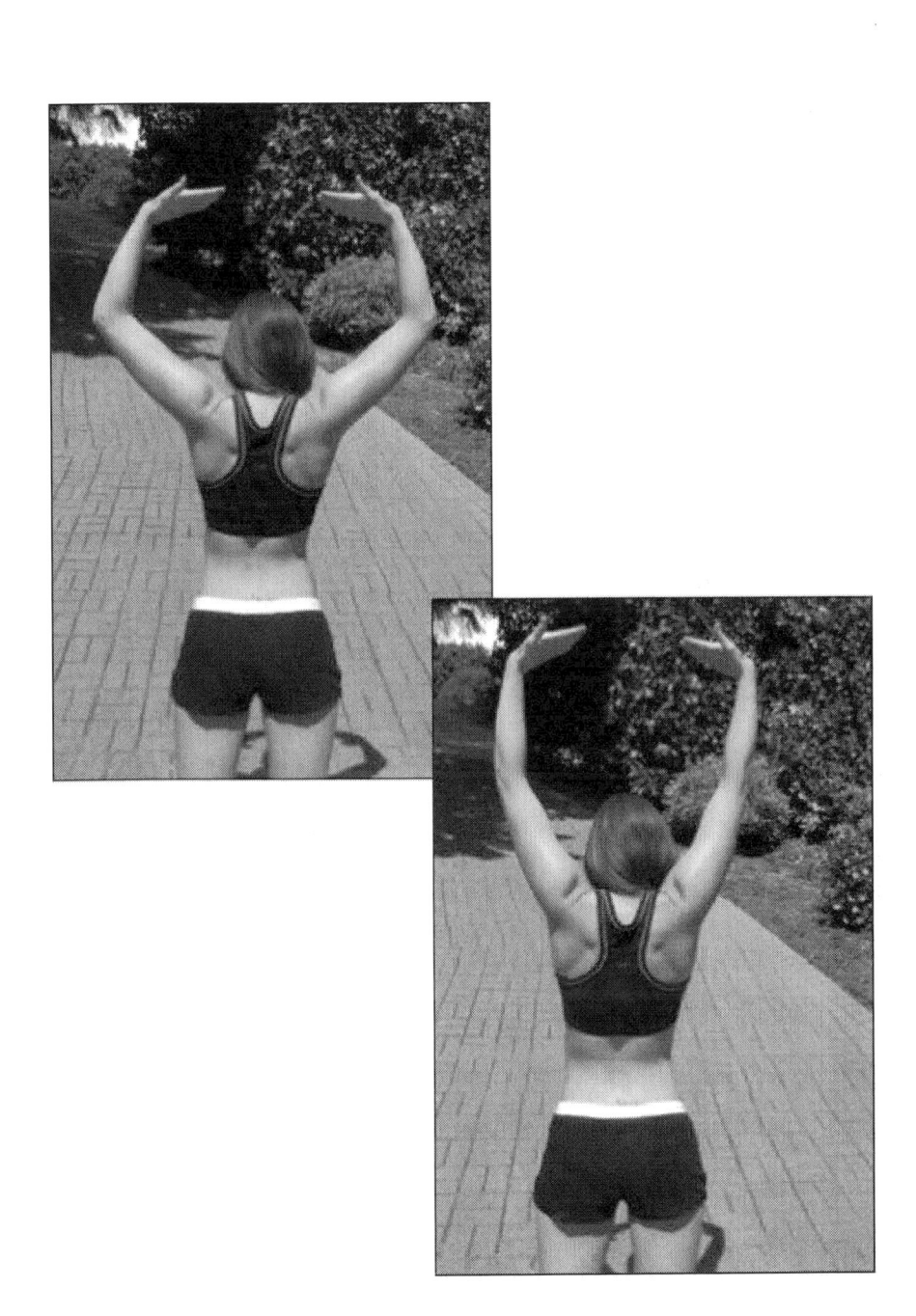

Gymnastic Shoulder Pulls

1. Begin with your feet shoulder width apart and your knees slightly bent.
2. Imagine that you are grabbing onto 2 buckets of water that you then lift up to your armpits.
3. From this position shrug your shoulders up so that they almost squeeze your head. Hold for a couple of seconds and release.
4. Repeat 10 times.

Additional Notes

- Primary areas worked - upper back, shoulder

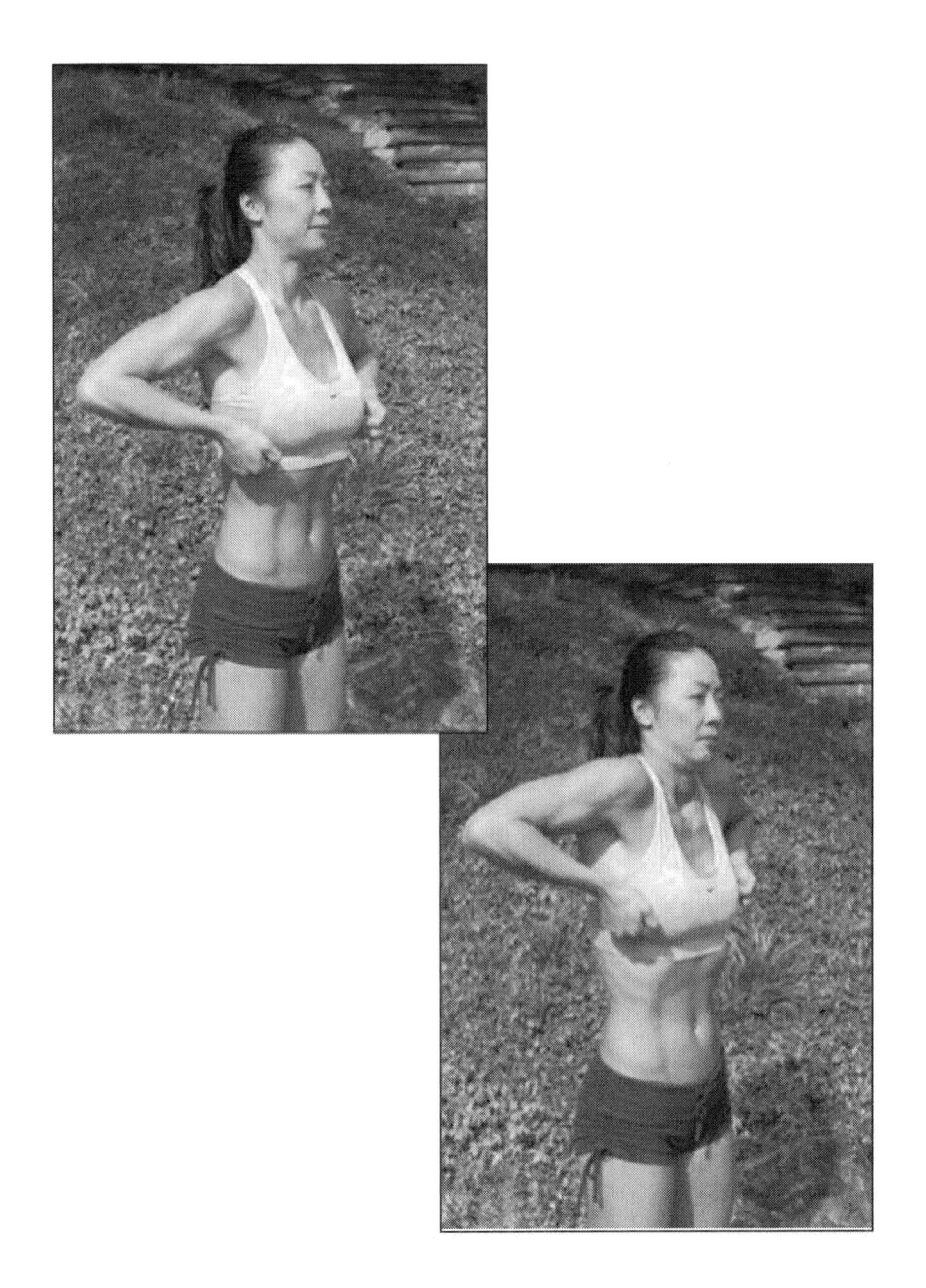

Gymnastic Shoulder Pulls 2

1. Begin with your feet shoulder width apart and your knees slightly bent.
2. Imagine that you are grabbing onto 2 buckets of water that you then lift up to your armpits.
3. From this position pinch your shoulders blades together by bringing your elbows back. Hold for a couple of seconds and release.
4. Repeat 10 times.

Additional Notes

- Primary areas worked - upper back, shoulder

77

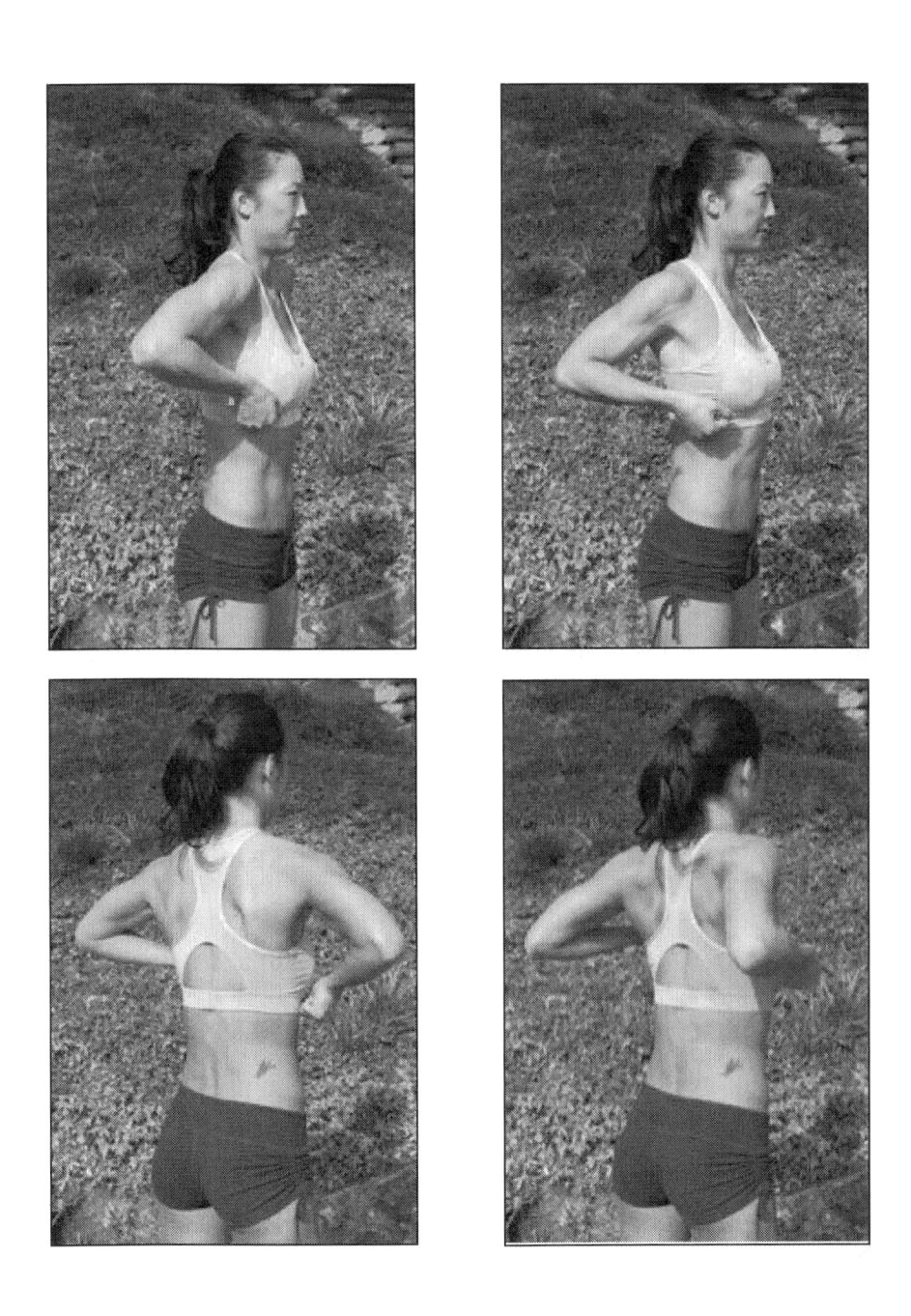

Towel Pulls

1. With your feet shoulder width apart and your knees slightly bent grab onto a towel that is approx. double your shoulder length apart.
2. Breathe in through your nose as you raise the towel above your head keeping your arms straight at all times.
3. Bring the towel behind you as you exhale your breathe through your nose.
4. Breathe in again and raise the towel above your head / exhale as you bring it in front of you.
5. Repeat 10 times.

Additional Notes

- Make sure you use a towel for this exercise as opposed to something with some give like rubber tubing.
- To begin you want to grab onto the towel with your hands as close together as possible while still allowing your arms to be straight when performing the movement. As you improve you will want to decrease this distance.
- Primary areas worked – shoulders, upper back

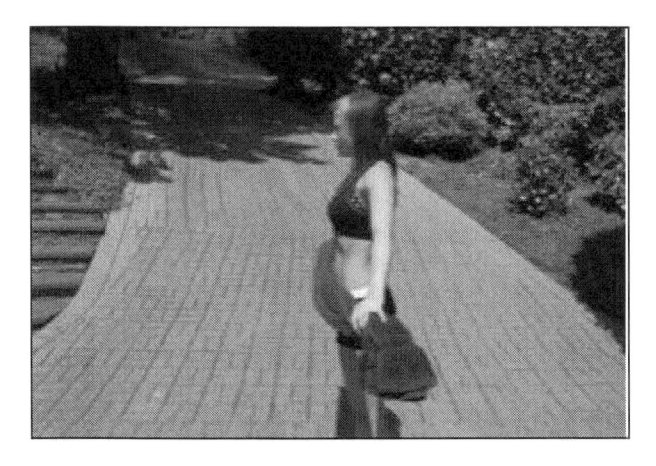

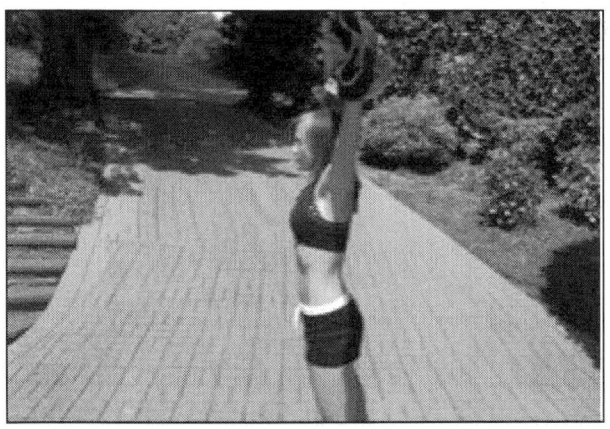

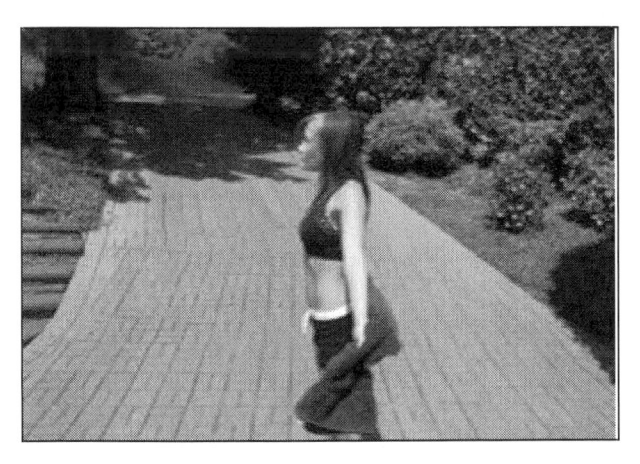

Side Towel Pulls

1. With your feet shoulder width apart and your knees slightly bent grab onto a towel that is approx. double your shoulder length apart.
2. With straight arms raise the towel above you head.
3. Pull to the right side using your right hand. This will force you to bend at the waist to the right.
4. Hold for a second then repeat on the opposite side.
5. Repeat 10 times.

Additional Notes

- Primary areas worked - upper back, shoulder, mid back

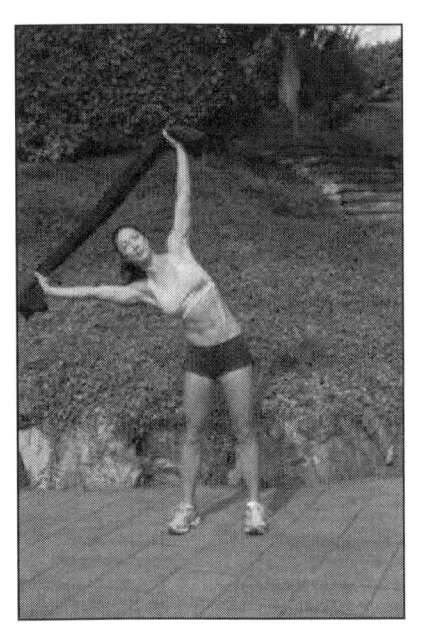

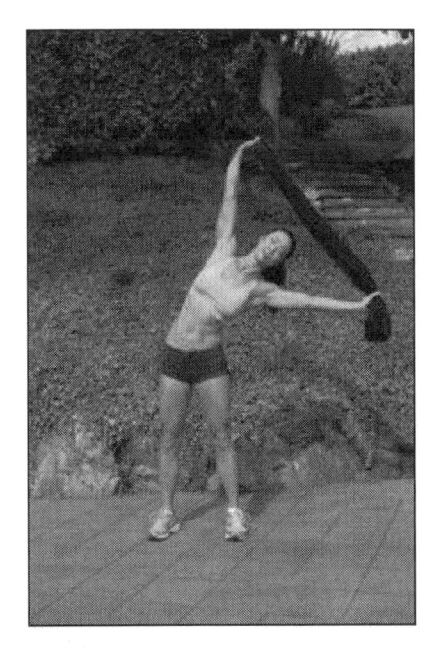

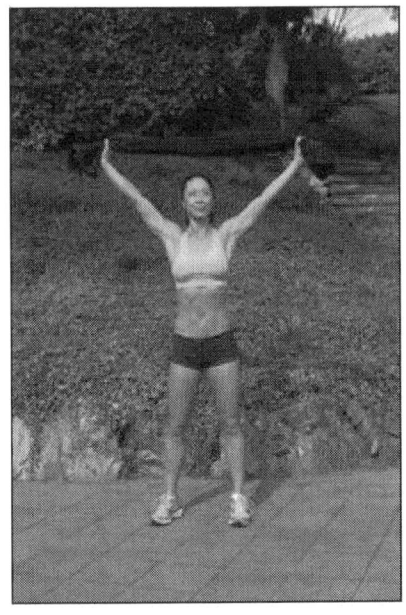

Dynamic Lion Stretch

1. Begin on all fours with your hands slightly wider than shoulder width in front of you and your feet double shoulder width behind you. Both your arms and legs should be straight.
2. Press back with your hands so that you are looking at a spot between your legs while keeping your back straight.
3. Keeping your arms and legs straight come forward so that you arch your back and you are looking at the ceiling.
4. Go back and forth like this 10 times.

Additional Notes

- This stretch is essentially a variation of a Hindu Pushup. The main difference is that you are keeping your arms straight.
- This is a great stretch for your shoulders, hips and spine.
- Primary areas worked - lower back, hips, shoulders

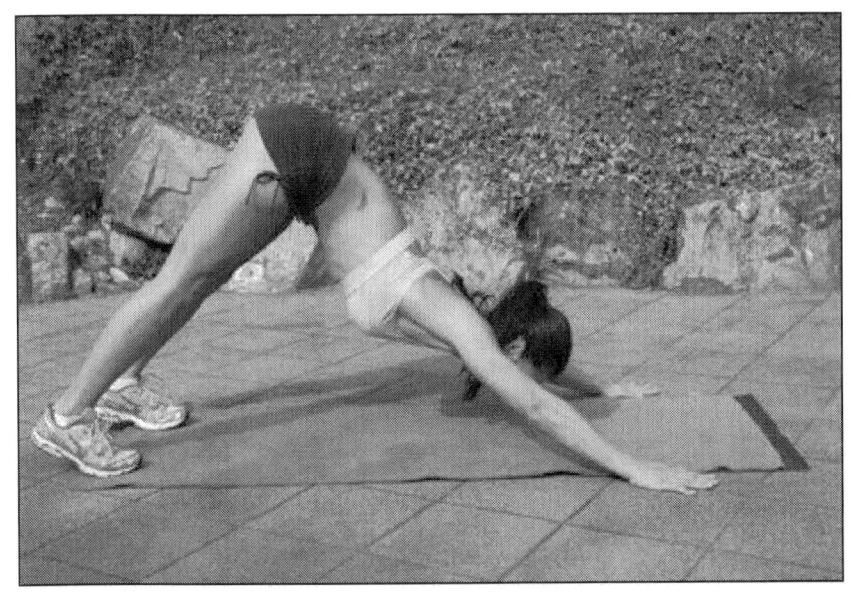

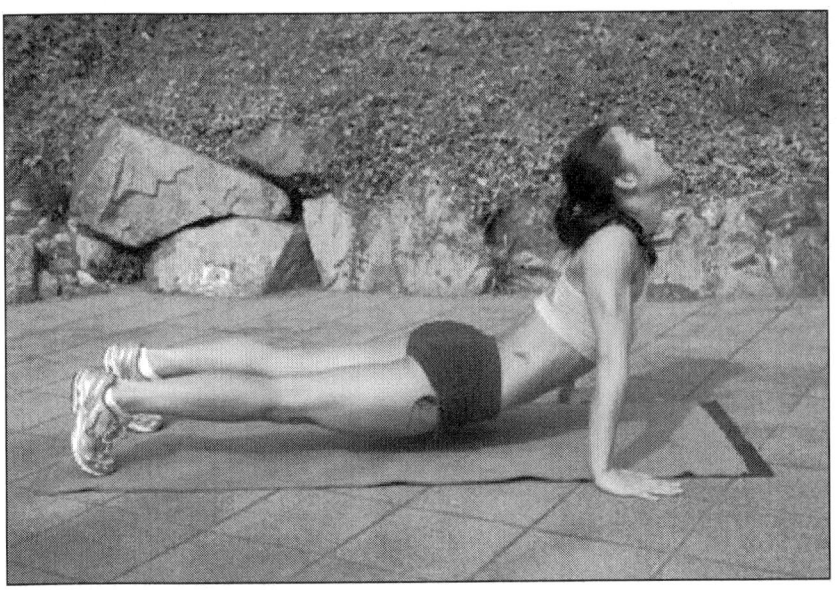

Kneeling Back Bend

1. Begin kneeling on the ground with your hips and pelvis forward.
2. Place your hands on your lower back and hips to support your lower back.
3. Look upwards as you bend at the knees backward as far as you can go.
4. Come back up.

Additional Notes

- This is a great stretch for your quads, hip flexors and lower back.
- Throughout this movement you will want to keep your hips, stomach and chest in a straight line. Do not cheat the movement by bending at the waist.
- When you get really good it is possible to bend so far back that your head touches the ground. If you can do this, great. Just remember again to not cheat the movement when you come up by bending at the waist.
- Primary areas worked - quadriceps, hips, lower back

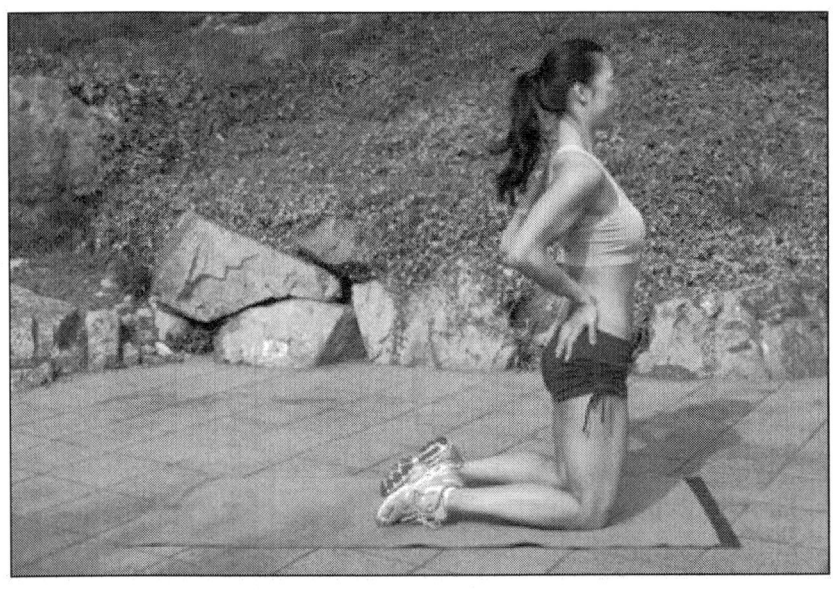

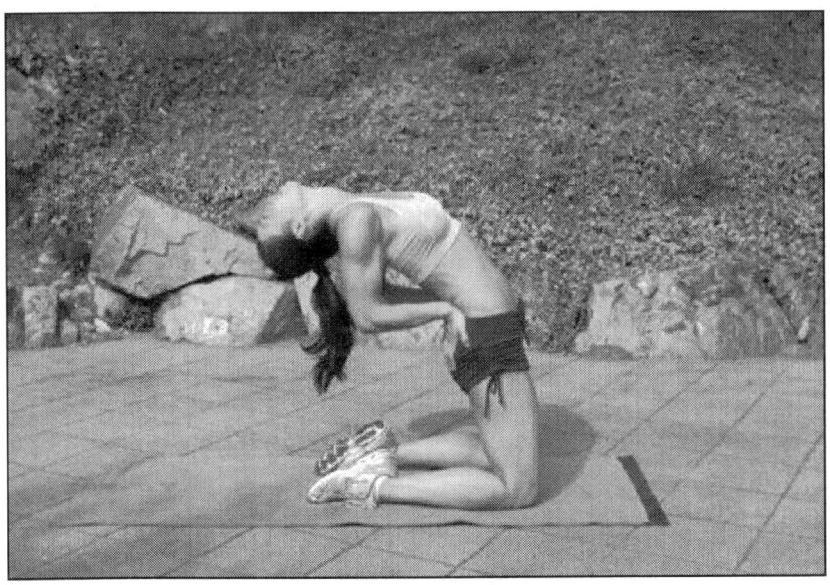

Forward Rows

1. Begin with your feet shoulder width apart.
2. Cross your forearms so that your palms are facing upwards and your wrists are parallel to each other.
3. Bend forward at the waist so that your arms are just below your waist. This is the starting position.
4. Exhale through your nose as you bend further at the waist bringing your arms towards the floor.
5. Inhale as you bend upwards at the waist again and you move back to the starting position.
6. Do this movement slowly. The result is a gentle rowing motion.
7. Repeat 10 times.

Additional Notes

- This is a great stretch for your hamstrings and lower back.
- If you have tight hamstrings bend your knees. This will relieve tension from the lower back.
- Never raise your back beyond parallel to the floor when performing this movement.
- Primary areas worked - hamstrings, lower back

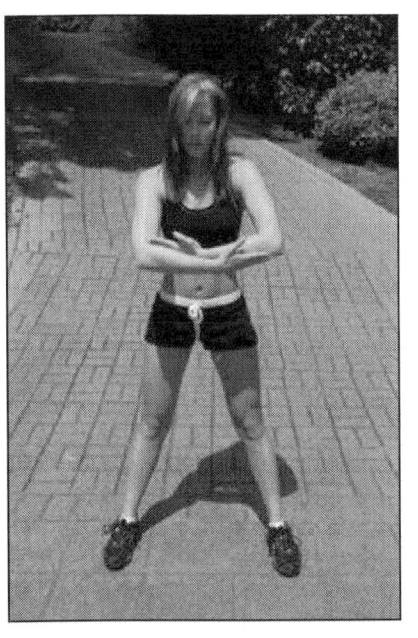

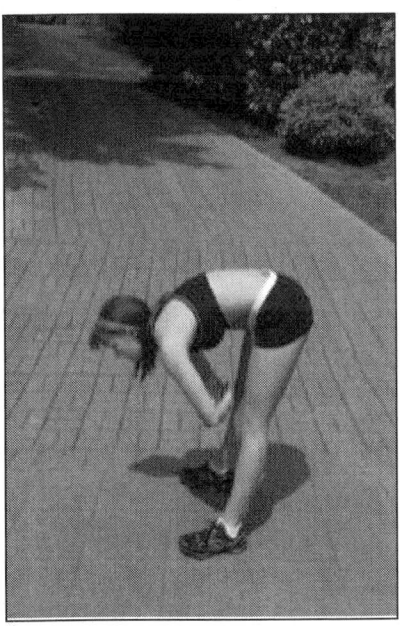

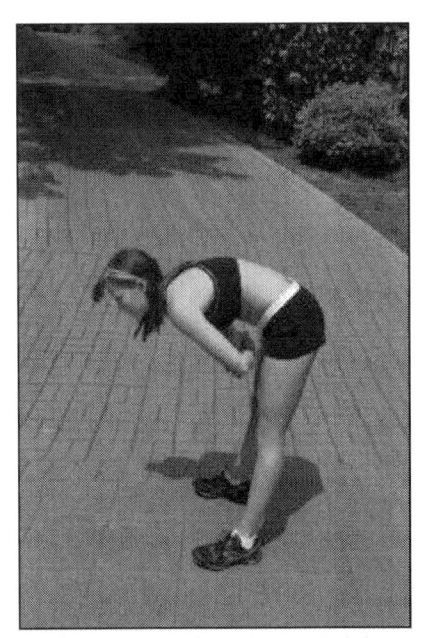

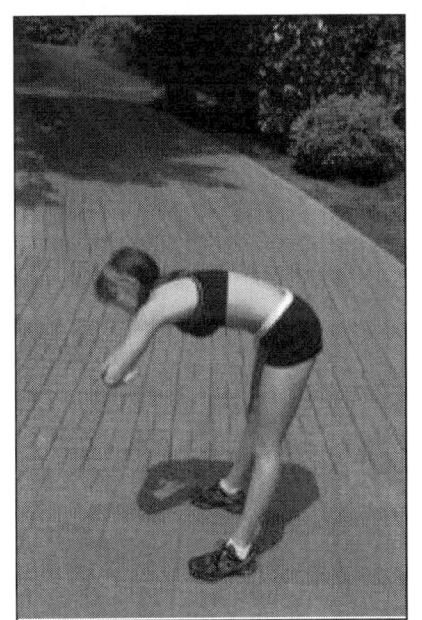

Hand Supported Back Bridge

This exercise is the same as the Dynamic Bridging Stretch, except this time you are holding it for time. Holding the Back Bridge for time may be the best exercise I know of to strengthen and stretch your back. Before attempting it I typically warm up with 10 Dynamic Bridge Stretches to warm up. I advise you to do the same.

1. Lie down on a soft mat with your back facing down.
2. Bend your legs so that your feet are close to your butt. Place your hands face down by your shoulders.
3. Pushup with your legs so that you arch your back, driving your body backwards. Your weight should now be supported by your feet, hands, and the top of your head.
4. Drive backwards with your feet so that your nose is touching the mat. Hold it there.
5. Breathe slowly and naturally through your nose. Concentrate on your breath, and try to remain as still as possible. This will make this exercise much easier.
6. Hold this position for as long as possible. If you can hold it for 1 minute you're doing great. Your ultimate goal, however, should be 3 minutes, which is the rough equivalent of 20 to 25 deep breaths.

Arms Folded Back Bridge

When you're comfortable performing the hand supported back bridge, you are ready to try it without hand support. The steps are the same as the above, except that now when you touch your nose to the mat, fold your arms in front of your chest. Again, shoot for three minutes, although you can really hold it for as long as you want.

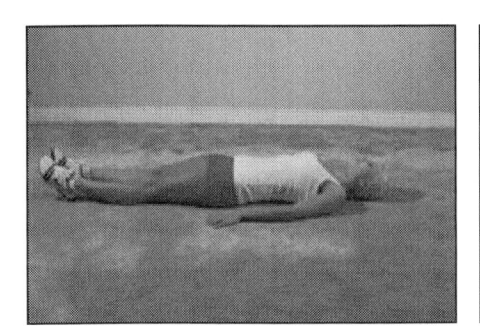

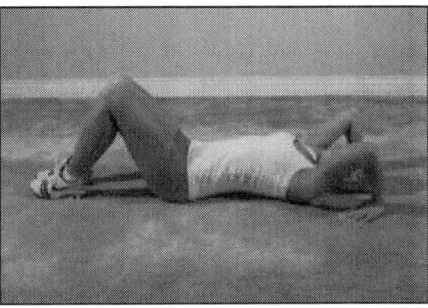

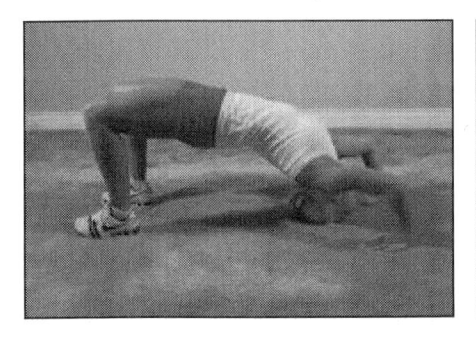

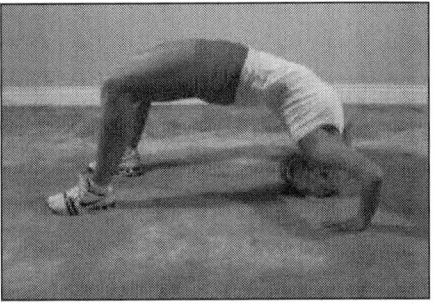

Floor Bow Posture

This is an exercise I learned in yoga. It really stretches and strengthens the muscles in your back, while increasing the flexibility of the spine.

1. Lie flat on the floor with your stomach on the ground.
2. Bend your legs backward so that you can grab the outside of your feet with your hands. Bend you head backwards so that you are looking at the ceiling.
3. Kick upwards and backwards with your legs. It is this force that will lift your legs and chest off the ground. You are not pulling on your feet with your hands. Think of them as ropes. They are simply there to prevent you from kicking your feet back to the ground.

Hold this position for about five slow, deep breaths.

91

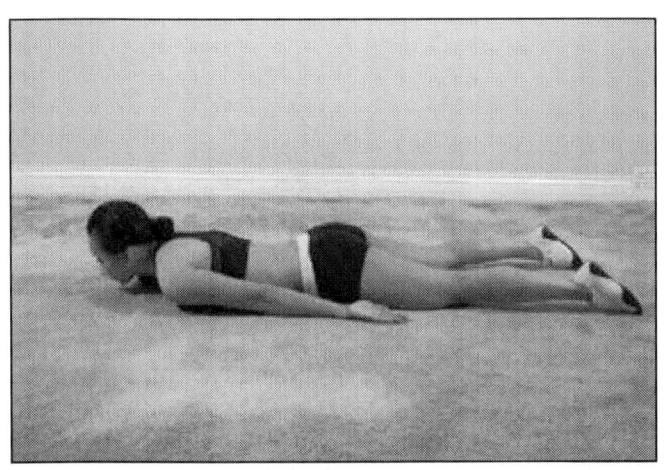

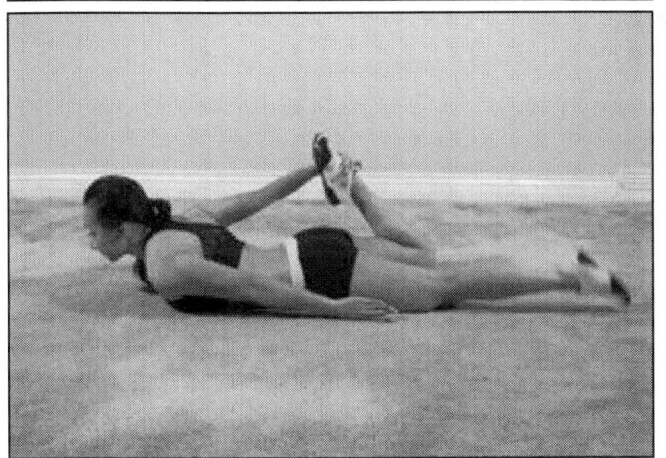

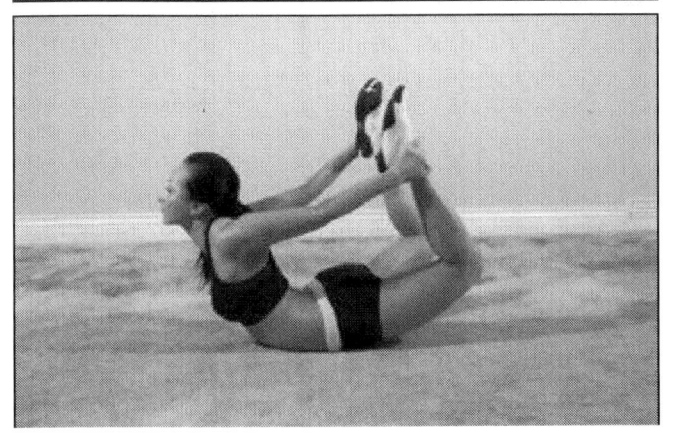

Wall Walking

This is another great exercise that really stretches your spine. When people start learning the back bridge this is often the exercise that they start with. The backward bending motion really works your abdominals, as they will be forced to contract. If you feel a twinge in your back after doing an activity like shoveling snow, a little wall walking is often just the thing to fix you up.

1. Stand with your heels and back flat against a bare wall.
2. Take three or four heel to toe steps forward from the wall. (As you get better at this exercise and improve your flexibility, you can take less).
3. Raise your hands upwards, palm towards the wall, and start to bend backwards.
4. Both hands should touch the wall with your fingertips pointing towards the floor.
5. Slowly walk your hands down the wall. This can feel very awkward at first. Just breathe deeply and calmly and work with gravity as your head approaches the floor.
6. Keep going until your forehead lightly touches the ground.

Once you are in this position you have a choice. You can either A) turn to your stomach and stand up again, or B) walk back up the wall with your hands.

Make sure you breathe naturally and slowly throughout this exercise. Five to Ten repetitions are usually plenty. After completing this exercise, it is often a good idea to stand and bend forward from the waist to stretch your spine in the opposite direction.

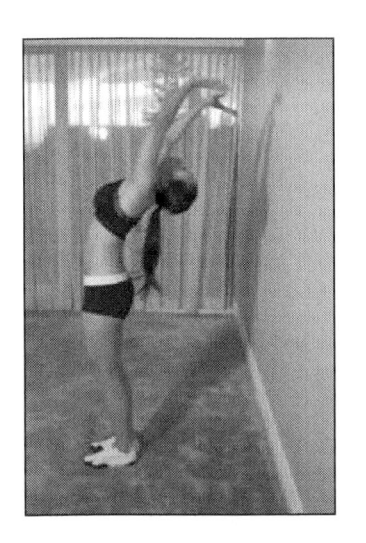

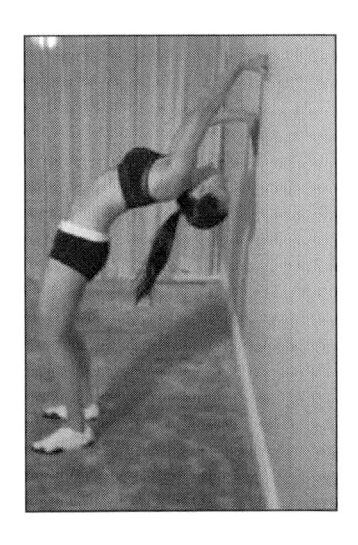

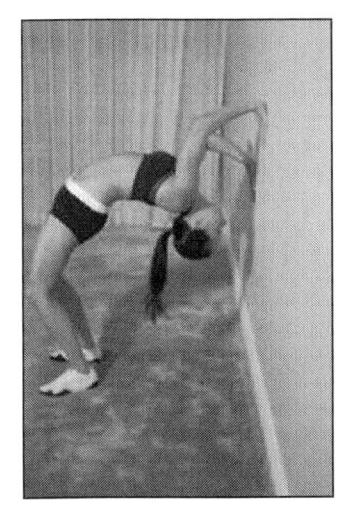

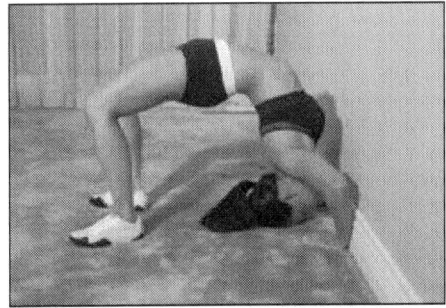

The Table Maker

Performing the table maker will promote flexibility in your spine while building strength in your back, triceps, shoulders, hips and buttocks.

1. Sit down on the floor with your feet straight in front of you and your back perpendicular to the floor.
2. Put the palms of your hands on the floor and push your body forward until the soles of your feet are flat on the ground. Arch your hips and back and let your head fall backward.
3. Squeeze your butt tightly as you straighten your back as much as you can. Your arms and lower legs should now be at 90-degree angles to your body and upper legs.
4. Hold yourself in this table position for a moment, and then lower yourself back to the starting position.

Try to perform 10 to 20 repetitions of this exercise. Inhale as you push yourself up, exhale on the downward motion.

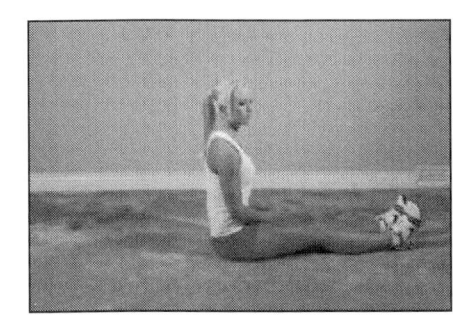

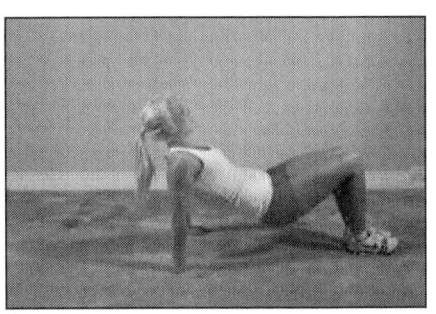

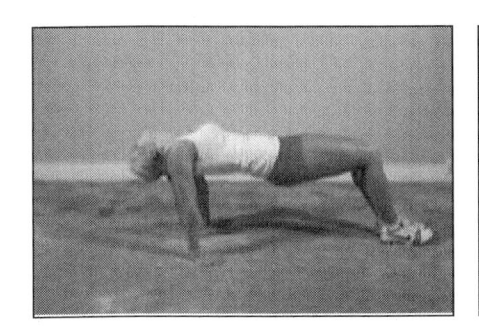

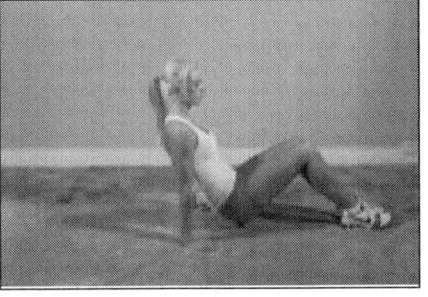

The Stretcher

This exercise is a more difficult variation of the table maker. When you've mastered the table maker, try the stretcher on for size.

1. Just like the table maker, sit on the floor with your legs out straight and your hands palm down at your sides.
2. Push your body forward so that your feet are flat on the ground while keeping your legs straight. Arch your hips and back. Keep both your legs and back as straight as possible.
3. Hold this position for a beat and then lower yourself gently to the floor.

You should aim to do 10 to 20 repetitions of this exercise. Inhale as you raise yourself up, exhale on the way down.

97

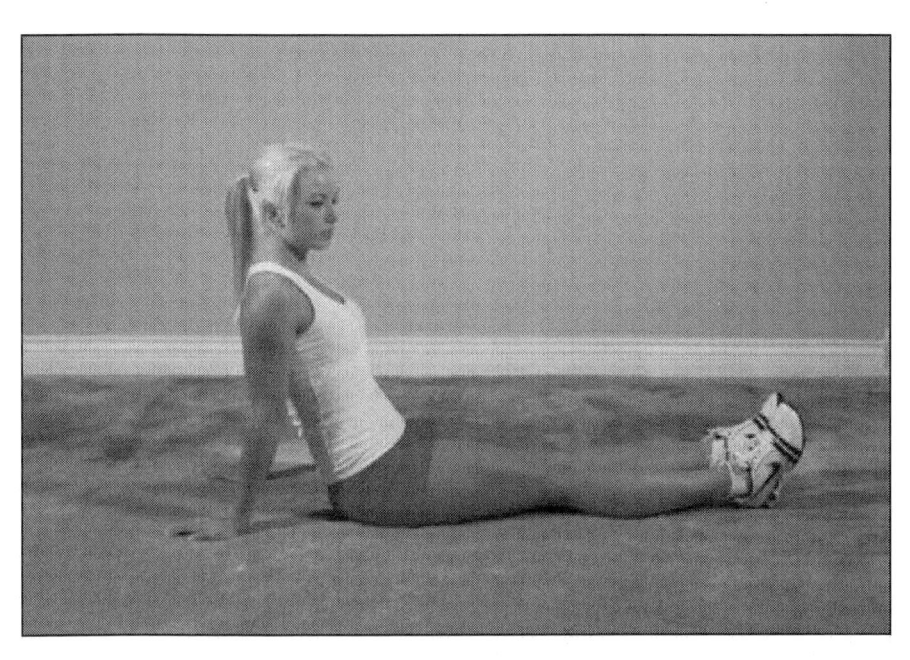

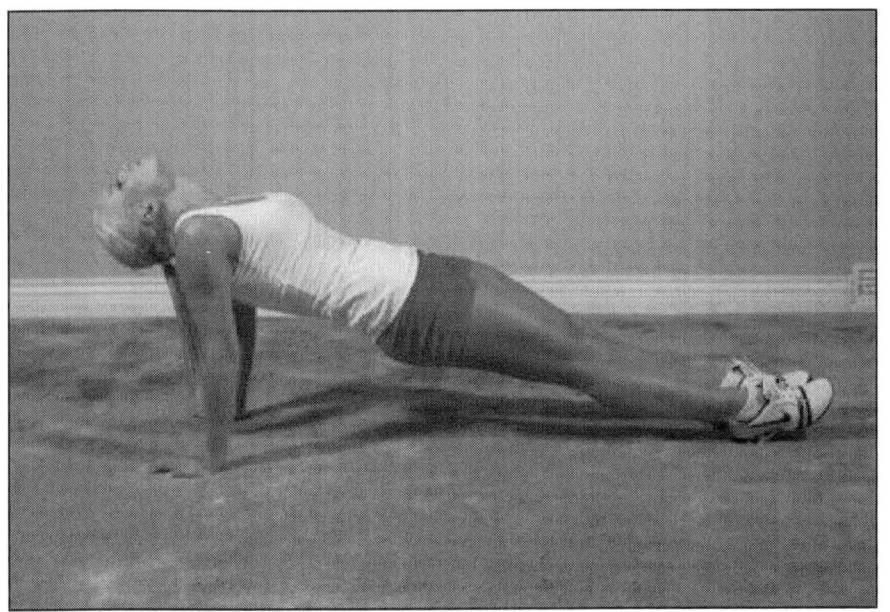

Reverse Leg Lifts

This exercise gives your lower back a good stretch. It also strengthens your abdominals, lower back, and buttocks.

1. Lie flat on the floor, face down, with your arms stretched forward.
2. Take a deep inhale and lift both legs at the same time. Hold for a couple of seconds.
3. Exhale your breath and lower your legs to the floor.

Keep you nose to the floor as you lift your legs in order to protect your back. You can bend your knees slightly if you wish.

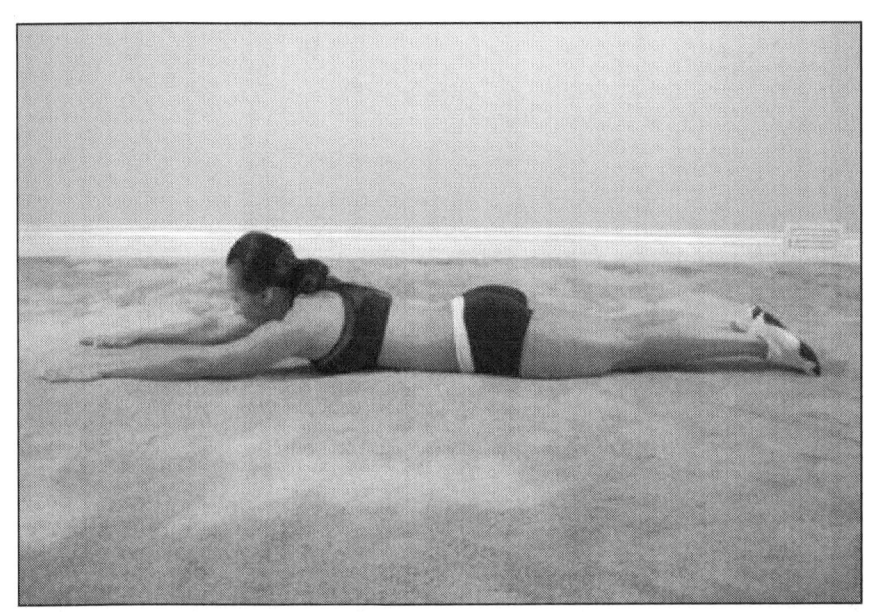

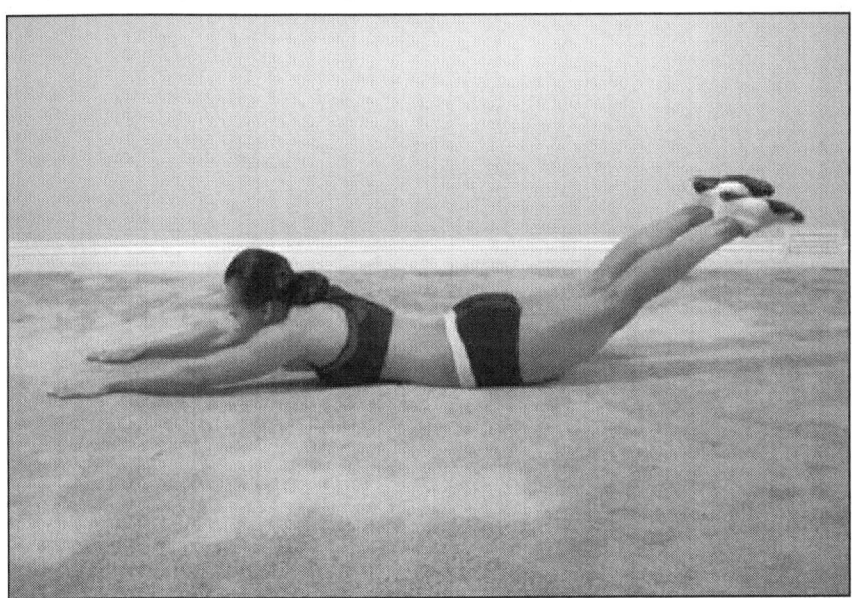

Torso Lifts

Torso lifts are the opposite of the leg lifts. You'll be surprised how much your abdominals, hips, and back are worked in this exercise. Plus, you get to pretend that you're Superman or Superwoman, which is kind of fun ;)

1. Lie face down on the floor with your arms stretched forward.
2. Keeping your legs on the ground, inhale and lift your arms, chest, and abdominals as high as you can. Hold for a second.
3. Exhale and lower yourself to the floor.

Try to perform this exercise 10 times at a minimum.

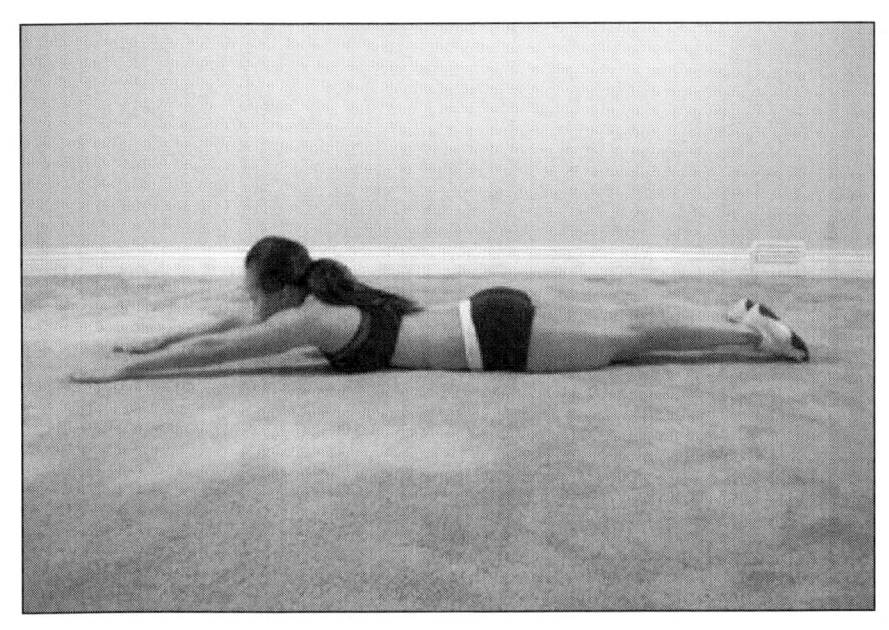

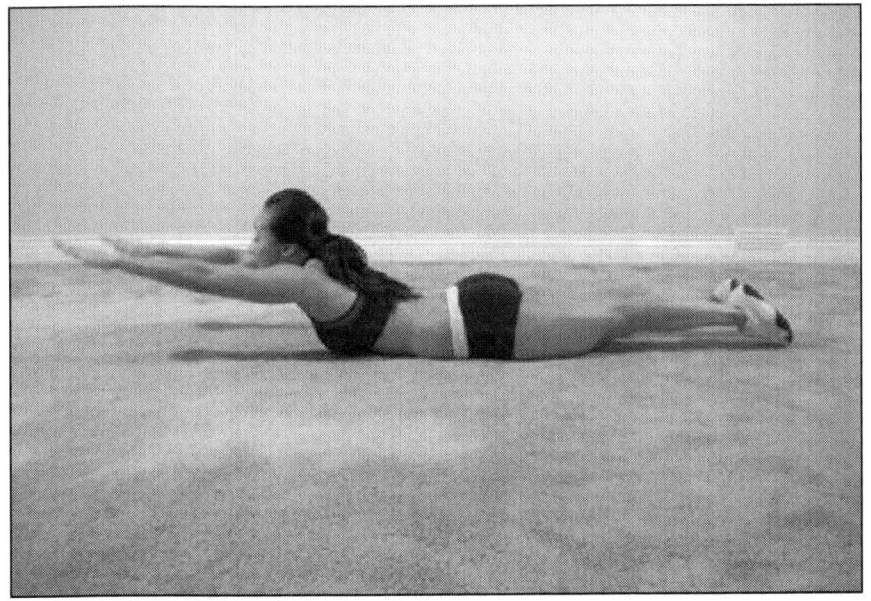

Isometric Neck Exercises

Reverse Neck Contraction

Position A

This exercise builds up the muscles in the back of the neck. There are 3 positions for this exercise. You can either do all three on one day or divide them up between 3 days.

1. Stand straight up with your knees slightly bent and your feet shoulder-width apart.
2. Make sure your abs are tucked in tight.
3. Keeping your spine straight, bend your neck forward so that your chin is tucked into your chest.
4. Clasp your hands together and place them behind your head.
5. Use your neck muscles to try and raise your head up as you resist with your clasped hands.
6. Remember to slowly increase the pressure by breathing in through the nose for 3 to 4 seconds.
7. When you've reached maximum tension in the neck exhale through your mouth for 7 to 12 seconds, making a "sssssss" sound as you do so.
8. Slowly release the tension in your neck while breathing in through your nose for another 3 to 4 seconds.

Position B

Repeat the steps for position A except this time begin with your neck straight so that it's inline with your spine. You should be looking straight ahead.

Position C

Repeat the steps for Position A except this time begin with your neck bent backwards so that you are looking up at the ceiling.

104

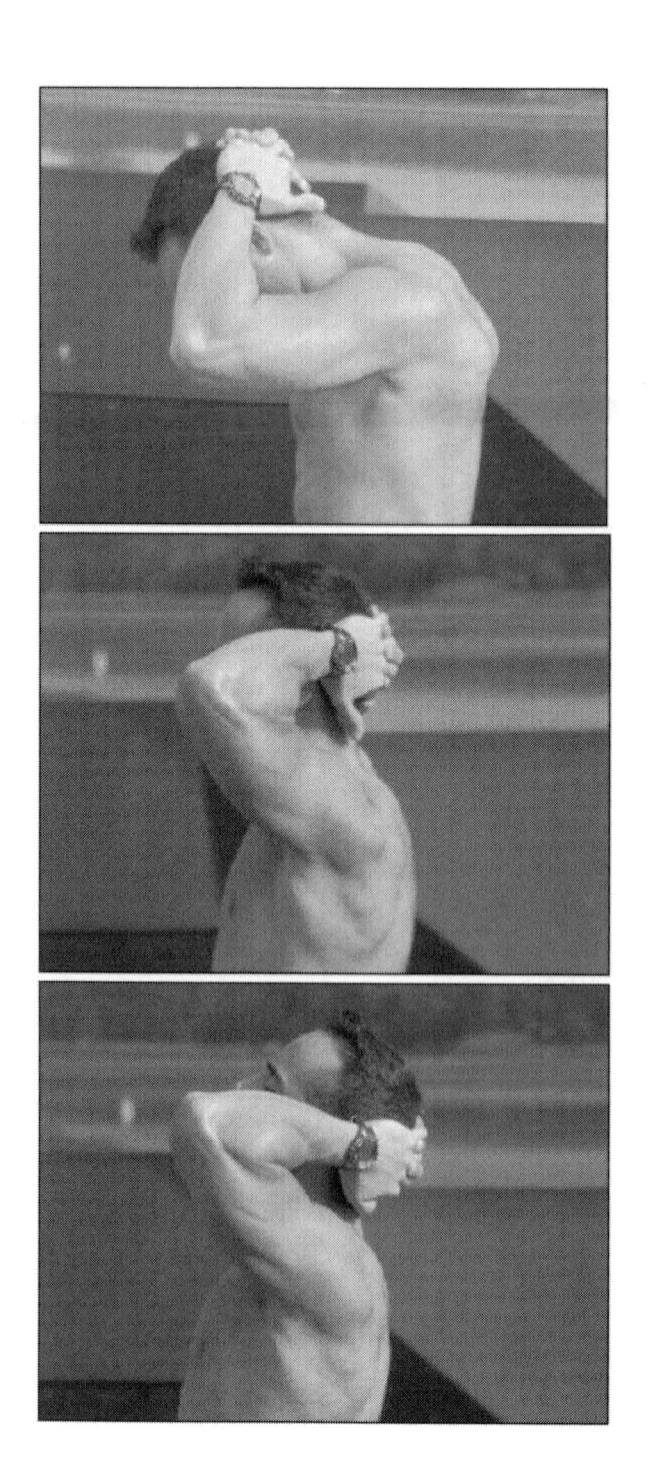

Forward Neck Contraction

Position A

This exercise builds up the muscles in the front of the neck. There are 3 positions for this exercise. You can either do all three on one day or divide them up between 3 days.

1. Stand straight up with your knees slightly bent and your feet shoulder-width apart.
2. Make sure your abs are tucked in tight.
3. Keeping your spine straight, bend your neck backward as far as you can.
4. Make your right hand into a fist and place it on your forehead with your thumb touching it. Clasp the top of your fist with your left hand.
5. Use your neck muscles to try and raise your head up as you resist with your hands.
6. Remember to slowly increase the pressure by breathing in through the nose for 3 to 4 seconds.
7. When you've reached maximum tension in the neck exhale through your mouth for 7 to 12 seconds, making a "sssssss" sound as you do so.
8. Slowly release the tension in your neck while breathing in through your nose for another 3 to 4 seconds.

Position B

Repeat the steps for position A except this time begin with your neck straight so that it's inline with your spine. You should be looking straight ahead.

Position C

Repeat the steps for Position A except this time begin with your head tilted forward with your chin touching your chest.

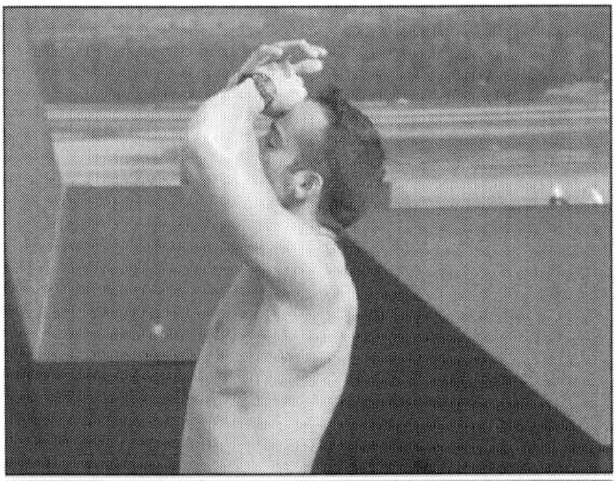
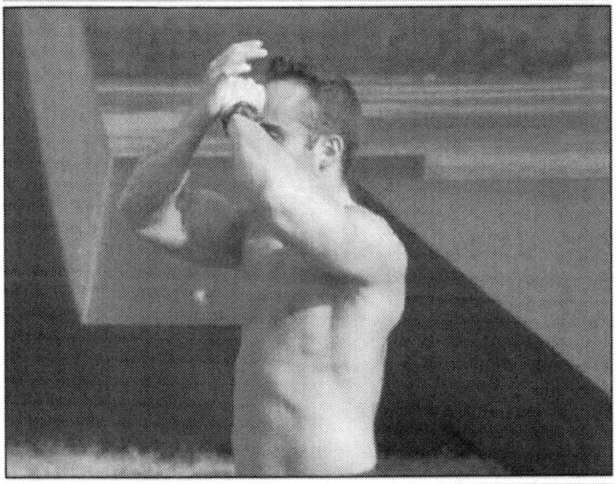
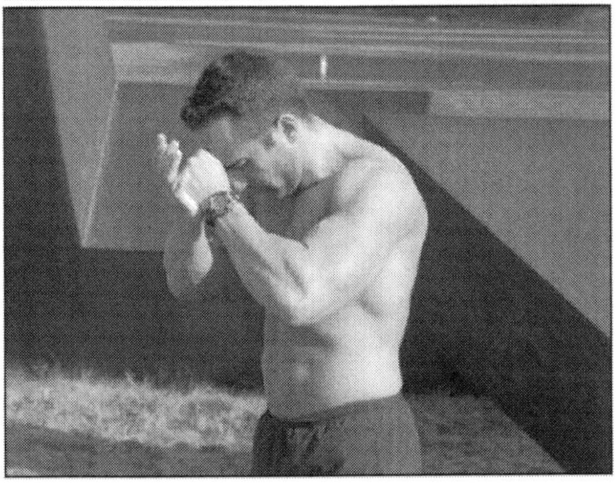

Side Neck Contraction (left to right)

Position A

This exercise builds up the muscles along the side of the neck. There are 3 positions for this exercise. You can either do all three on one day or divide them up between 3 days.

1. Stand straight up with your knees slightly bent and your feet shoulder-width apart.
2. Make sure your abs are tucked in tight.
3. Keeping your spine straight, tilt your head towards your left shoulder.
4. Place your right hand on the right side of your head for resistance.
5. Use your neck muscles to try and raise your head up from your left shoulder as you resist with your right hand.
6. Remember to slowly increase the pressure by breathing in through the nose for 3 to 4 seconds.
7. When you've reached maximum tension in the neck exhale through your mouth for 7 to 12 seconds, making a "sssssss" sound as you do so.
8. Slowly release the tension in your neck while breathing in through your nose for another 3 to 4 seconds.

9.

Position B

Repeat the steps for position A except this time begin with your neck straight so that it's inline with your spine.

Position C

Repeat the steps for Position A except this time begin with your neck tilted towards your right shoulder.

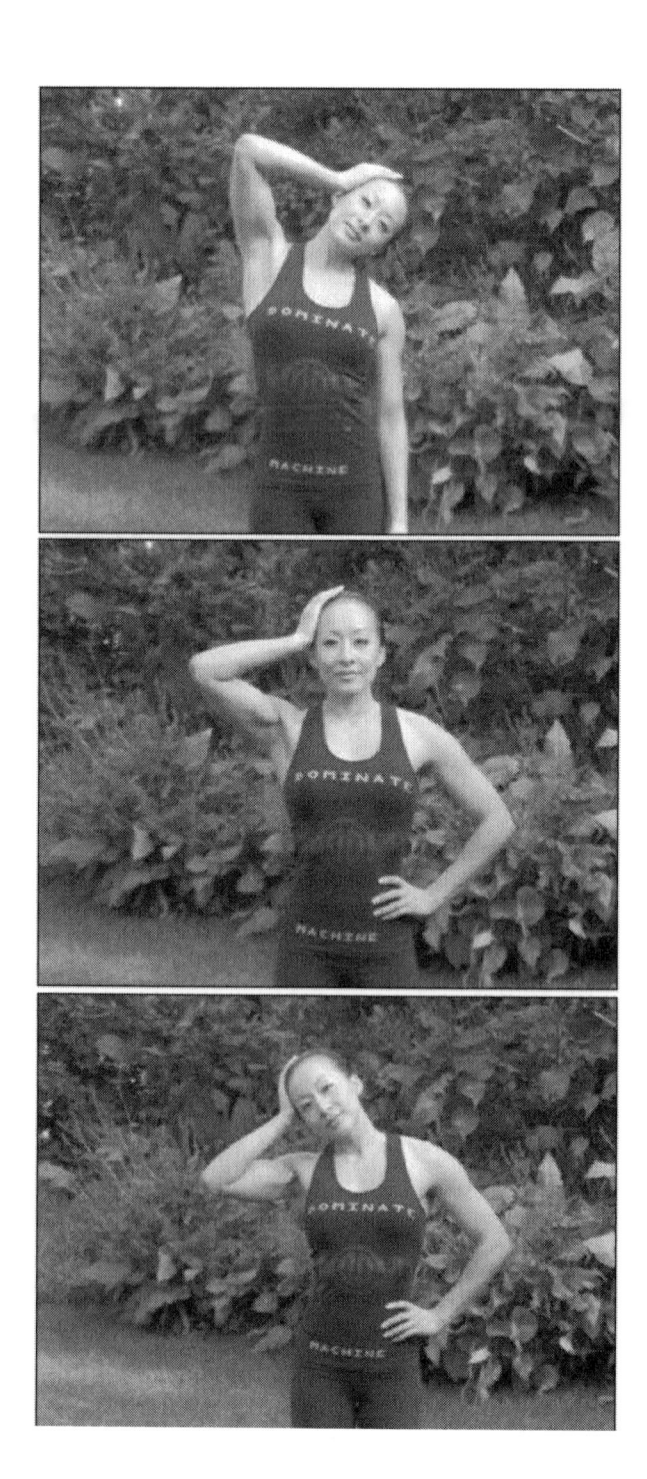

Side Neck Contraction (right to left)

Position A

This exercise builds up the muscles along the opposite side of the neck. There are 3 positions for this exercise. You can either do all three on one day or divide them up between 3 days.

1. Stand straight up with your knees slightly bent and your feet shoulder-width apart.
2. Make sure your abs are tucked in tight.
3. Keeping your spine straight, tilt your head towards your right shoulder.
4. Place your left hand on the left side of your head for resistance.
5. Use your neck muscles to try and raise your head up from your right shoulder as you resist with your left hand.
6. Remember to slowly increase the pressure by breathing in through the nose for 3 to 4 seconds.
7. When you've reached maximum tension in the neck exhale through your mouth for 7 to 12 seconds, making a "ssssss" sound as you do so.
8. Slowly release the tension in your neck while breathing in through your nose for another 3 to 4 seconds.

Position B

Repeat the steps for position A except this time begin with your neck straight so that it's inline with your spine.

Position C

Repeat the steps for Position A except this time begin with your neck tilted towards your right shoulder.

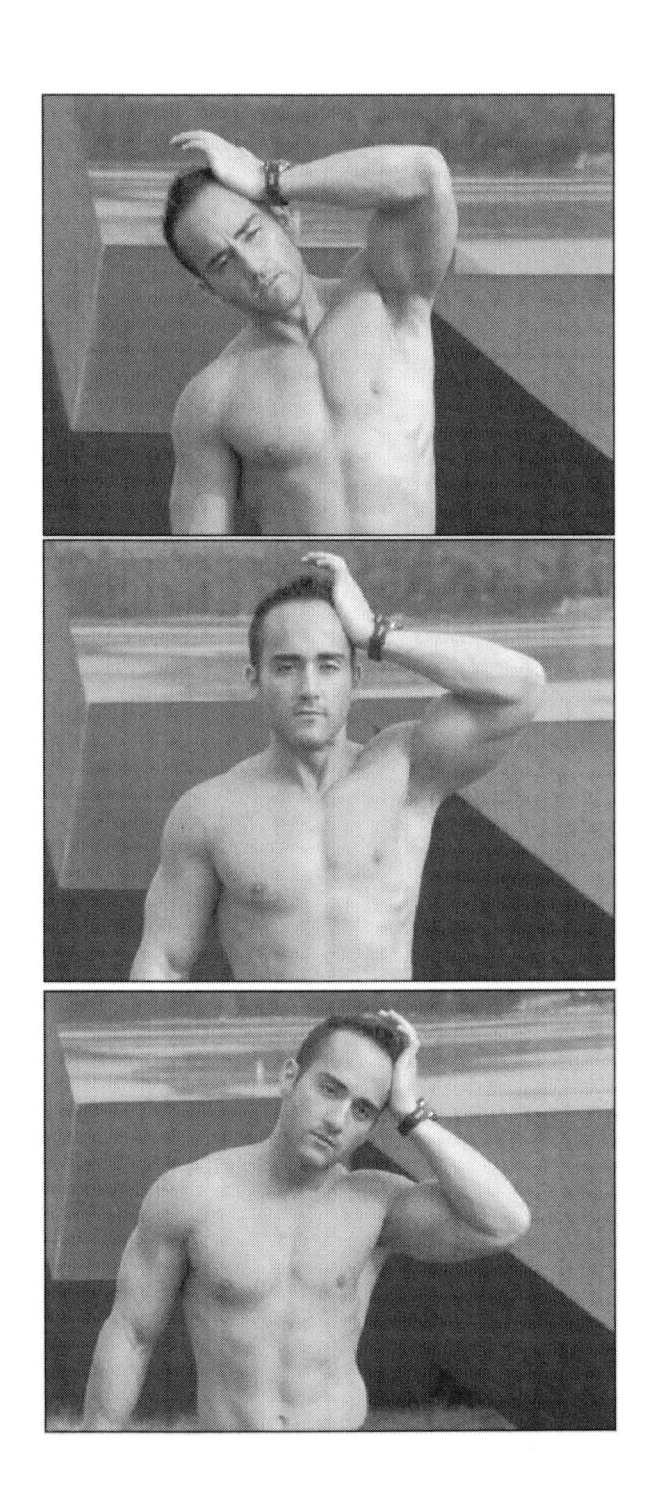

Suggested Back Stretching And Strengthening Routines

Taking A Break From Sitting Stretches

A great many of us work at jobs which require us to sit for long periods of time. If you are able or if you feel the need, it is highly advisable to stand for a few minutes and do one of two of the following stretches. They will invigorate you and your back will thank-you for it.

Standing Back Rotation Stretch
Grounded Back Twist
Tai Chi Waist Turner

Beginner Back Stretching and Strengthening Routine

Tai Chi Waist Turner
Ying/Yang Bends
Neck Stretch
Reverse Neck Contraction
Forward Neck Contraction
Side Neck Contraction (left to right)
Side Neck Contraction (right to left)
Reverse Leg Lifts
Torso Lifts

Intermediate Back Stretching and Strengthening Routine

Tai Chi Waist Turner
Grounded Back Twist

Dynamic Lion Stretch
Cobra Stretch
4 Point Neck Stretch
Reverse Neck Contraction
Forward Neck Contraction
Side Neck Contraction (left to right)
Side Neck Contraction (right to left)
The Table Maker

Advanced Back Stretching and Strengthening Routine

Tai Chi Waist Turner
Grounded Back Twist
Forward Rows
Kneeling Back Bend
Reverse Neck Contraction
Forward Neck Contraction
Side Neck Contraction (left to right)
Side Neck Contraction (right to left)
Table Maker Stretch
Dynamic Bridging Stretch
Hand Supported Back Bridge

Stretching Routine For Lower Back Tension

Although this stretching routine can be done anytime, I've found it is particularly effective if done right before bedtime.

Lying Groin Stretch
Knee To Shoulder Stretch
Shoulder Blade Pinch

Lower Back Flattener
Neck Stretch
Secretary Stretch
Lying Groin Stretch (repeated)
Secretary Stretch (repeated)
Elongation Stretch
Cobra Stretch
Double Knee To Chest Stretch

Intramuscular Stimulation

I presume the reason you bought this book (and thank-you for doing so!) is that you, like most people, have had issues with back pain and discomfort in the past. The whole reason I have spent so much time in the past researching and trying different back stretching and strengthening methods was to deal with my own back pain. In this final section I want to tell you my story of back pain, as well as a relatively new technique that was used to basically cure me. I'm including it here as, although it is a technique you would have to consult a qualified physiotherapist to experience, I think it might really help you. Here's my story.

For many years I lifted weights at Gold's Gym. On one occasion I was doing a leg press when I felt something move in my back. Actually, it felt much worse than that. It felt like bones and muscles that don't normally move suddenly jumped and then settled again. Although I remained calm on the outside, on the inside I was freaking out. Would I be able to move?

Would some bodybuilders have to come over and pick me up so that I could go to a hospital? I was really concerned.

Lucky for me, I was able to move under my own steam, although very slowly. I had definitely done a number on my back, but time heals all wounds right? Being young and stupid (you always feel that you're invincible when you're young) I didn't even bother to see a doctor. I just let nature take its course. Idiot.

Over the next two weeks my back did get better, but it was never 100%. From then on my lower back was always tight. What's worse, this manifested itself in my calves always being constricted as well. When I got up in the morning my calves would be so tight I had to stretch them just so that they would feel OK. I knew that my back wasn't quite right, but I had no idea how to fix it.

This is what started me on my back strengthening and stretching journey. I read a ton of books, and tried just about every therapy out there. Although the exercises in this book completely helped me strengthen and stretch my back (the stretching routine before going to bed was a particular godsend), I was always aware that I wasn't quite getting at the root of the issue. It was like the default state for my back was tightness. Why was this? Everything I did only seemed to manage the issue. I was never able to fix it.

In addition, usually once a year, my back would just blow up. My back muscles would spasm and I'd be lying flat on the floor for days. I almost took this for granted. It was just something that happens. Accept it, deal with it, and move on. The last time (and now I'm hoping it IS the last time) this happened to me I was vacuuming out my car. I could tell that my back was bothering me a bit, but I had things I had to do, so I ignored it. As I was bending and turning awkwardly, BAM, there goes my back! That's what you get for ignoring your body. Looks like I had a date with my floor and bad daytime TV. How much does this suck?

Except this time it didn't. This time I had some new information.

From a friend, I learned about this technique I had never heard of called "Intramuscular Stimulation". This person, who had it done, was raving about it. Apparently, people were flying in from New York and LA just to have it done here in Vancouver by a man named Colin Miller. Intrigued, I had filed this away in the back of my brain. Now that I couldn't move, I thought I'd give it a shot.

Intramuscular Stimulation is essentially an outgrowth of acupuncture. People may disagree with me, but I see it as a westernized, more intense version of this ancient technique. The idea behind it is that our muscles are controlled by our nerves. When our muscles experience stress it is the nerves that send out signals to contract or relax. However, sometimes we can put so much trauma on our muscles (for example, doing leg presses with too much weight) that our nerves become stressed as well. They stop sending out the signal to relax and our muscles stay tight. I suspect this is what happened with my permanently tight back.

Intramuscular Stimulation attempts to fix this condition my re-stressing the nerves. This is accomplished by placing needles into the muscles. This forces the nerves to send out intense contraction signals to the muscle. When the outside trauma, in this case the needles, are removed, the nerves send out equally intense relaxation signals. In my mind it's almost like rebooting a computer. The trauma the needles produce allows the nerves to reset to "factory standard", if you will.

When I had this done the results were almost instantaneous. Right away I could tell something was different. Not only could I now walk around but I could tell that this technique was getting at the root of my back issues. Over the next 5 sessions I basically restored my back to the way it was prior to my weight lifting accident. Combine this with the back stretching and strengthening exercises I had already learned and my back had never felt better. Amazing!

Is there a downside to this technique? Well, yes. It is painful. The needles used here are much larger than the ones used for acupuncture. When the needles go in you will feel it. However, the pain is bearable. The question you have to ask yourself, if you're contemplating this treatment, is can I put up with 10 minutes of pain in order to experience long-term gain? For me the answer was obvious, and this is from a guy who hates getting flu shots. If I can do it, so can you.

If you're interested in this technique, check out Colin's website here:

http://www.sportandspinal.com/

Please note that I am getting no financial compensation for this. I am merely providing this information because it has helped me, and it might be helpful to you too, depending on your situation.

If you are interested in Intramuscular Stimulation, but you don't live in Vancouver, I suggest you "use the Google" to find a practitioner in your area. My only words of advice are that you want to find someone who is aggressive. What can happen is that an individual will advertise that they offer IMS treatment. However, when they perform the procedure, they may only stick you with 4 or 5 needles. I suspect that the issue here is that people who get involved in physical therapy want to help and heal people. However, when they try using IMS they are initially causing their patient some short-term pain and discomfort, causing them to back off too soon. This reaction is understandable, but unfortunate. If you're like me, you want to be fixed as soon as possible. Colin would stick me with between 20 and 30 needles at a time, for example.

Again, I've only brought this up because IMS really helped relieve my extreme back issues. If your back issues are more typical, the stretches and strengthening exercises in this book should suffice. Only you know what condition your spine is ultimately in and what techniques will benefit you. What you need is information. In this book I have attempted to give you as much as I can, based on my own journey dealing with back pain.

In yoga there is a saying that a healthy spine equals a happy life. I believe this is very true. When your spine is limber and youthful, you will be limber and youthful as well. Acquiring and maintaining a strong and healthy spine is worth the effort. I sincerely hope this book helps you get there.

If you have any questions about this book or the stretching exercises contained within it, feel free to contact me through my fitness website at animal-kingdom-workouts.com. Use the contact form. I appreciate all feedback, as this is the only way I know of to make my books better. Thank-you again and good luck to you!

About the Author

David Nordmark has a life long interest in health and fitness. In the past he has participated in such sports as soccer, basketball and hockey. He also was once an avid runner and weightlifter, but has since come to his senses. Today he mainly does natural exercises like Yoga and the Body Weight exercises found on his website, www.animal-kingdom-workouts.com.

He currently lives in beautiful Vancouver, British Columbia Canada, although he really wouldn't mind living somewhere else during the winter. He's currently working on making that dream a reality.

If you have any questions for him, feel free to contact him using the contact form which can be found on this website. Here's the link: http://www.animal-kingdom-workouts.com/contactme.html

About the Models

Christine Chou is a Vancouver-based fitness competitor. She can be reached at chrischou_@hotmail.com or through her website at

http://fitfabfoodies.com/

Bry Jensen is a university student and fitness model based in Abbotsford, British Columbia, Canada. She can be reached through her website at

http://www.bryjensen.com/

To view her modelling portfolio vist

http://www.modelmayhem.com/1341216

Sean Stewart is a specialized personal fitness trainer and fitness consultant. Sean also does coaching, acting, fitness modeling and online marketing. You may contact him by email at fitmanfrombc@gmail.com or through his website at

www.SeanFitness.com.

Kerry Diotte is a Vancouver-based model who enjoys exercise and playing soccer. She is available for fitness, glamour, and commercial modeling work. She can be reached at kerrydiotte05@msn.com. To view her portfolio, visit

http://www.modelmayhem.com/633989.

Karen Pang is a Vancouver-based fitness model and competitor. She also travels frequently to Los Angeles and Toronto. She is available for fitness modeling, glamour and bikini shoots. She can be reached at karen@misskarenpang.com or through her website at www.misskarenpang.com. To view her portfolio, visit

http://www.modelmayhem.com/558190

One Last Thing

When you turn the page, Kindle will give you the opportunity to rate the book and share your thoughts through an automatic feed to your Facebook and Twitter accounts. If you believe your friends would get something valuable out of this book, I'd be honored if you'd post your thoughts. As well, if you liked the book, I'd be eternally grateful if you posted a review on Amazon. Thank-you once again and I hope you enjoyed the book!

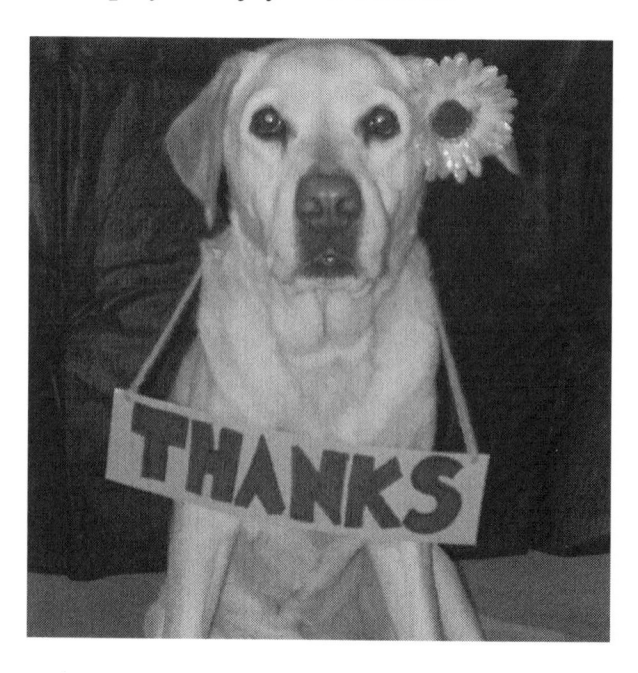

Printed in Great Britain
by Amazon.co.uk, Ltd.,
Marston Gate.